9 Easy Weightloss Tricks

Author: Mele Maja Faifaiumu
Isbn : 978-969-2992-48-0

ABOUT THE BOOK

Assuming you've been battling with your weight for some time, you'll realize that shedding those undesirable pounds and keeping them off can challenge. To supercharge your weight-reduction plan, Keep your health improvement plan on target by following these straightforward tips to eat less, consume more calories, and shed pounds.

Might you want to shed pounds rapidly and without any problem? Then, at that point, this book is for you!
These 9 simple weight reduction stunts will assist you with shedding 10 pounds right away.

"Nine of the Simplest Weight reduction Stunts" is a book loaded with tips and deceives to help the people who are struggling with losing those additional weight. This book will direct you with data on the most proficient method to lose those loads and lose them quick!

TABLE OF CONTENT

INTRODUCTION

Without question, anybody can get their hands on weight reduction materials. It's simple. It's all over the place. The battle confronted isn't such a great amount about getting the material on weight reduction or attempting to circle back to what is written in the book, yet rather seeing the progressions that you want without avoiding the arrangement with regard to dissatisfaction, having attempted the arrangement. For such a long time! Might you at any point relate? I suspected as much.

All things considered, consider the possibility that I let you know that in under multi month, you could lose 10 lbs by following 9 simple weight reduction stunts.

Indeed, you reserve each privilege to be mindful, given the numerous strategies you've attempted and the many eating regimens you've followed. In any case, I comprehend how it seems like to feel stuck and not lose the weight you want. That feeling when nothing is by all accounts working even in the wake of making a solid attempt. I have not come here to burn through your time or give you ridiculous expectations and make you put forth unattainable objectives, NO!

As a single parent (with simply a girl) who loves finding out about weight reduction, I have come to find during that time that the explanation your weight reduction venture has been a battle is that you have considered your weight to be an extremely perplexing issue that needs a complicated way to deal with prevail. In any case, as a general rule, this approach has never appeared to work. Because of my endometriosis torment, I was unable to practice that much, yet I've attempted a great deal of eating less junk food and expert methods to assist with getting more fit with practically no progressions until I tracked down these nine straightforward stunts. I call them the bypasses for weight reduction! I would like you to foster a methodology that is not difficult to achieve and, all the more significantly, reasonable.

The easiest and most reasonable method for keeping a solid weight is by counting calories. While this doesn't sound as marvelous or as in vogue as numerous different eating regimens, what it has making it work is that it's worked and will keep on working for a very

Long time. Assume you eat a larger number of calories than you consume and your weight increments. On the off chance that you eat similar measure of calories as you consume, your weight remains something similar. The more calories you eat, the less you consume, and your weight diminishes — and that is our objective. By simply following the stunts in this book, you can diminish the calories you take and furthermore all the while increment the calories you consume.

Getting more fit utilizing these stunts requires change, however it doesn't need to be troublesome. The thought is to fool your body into feeling happy with less calories and furthermore get to consume more calories. All through this book, we will follow this straightforward equation: Consume a bigger number of calories than you take in. To keep the numerical straightforward, our objective all through each stunt is to help you eat less and consume more!

However long you follow the stunts from this book, you'll find weight reduction can be simple. Rather than going for the stars and going for sensational and excruciating weight reduction, we're picking something reasonable so we can change your way of life. Rather than being on a tight eating routine, this way of life essentially becomes what your identity is.

The most awesome aspect of this book is that you just have to completely focus on a modest bunch of the stunts I'll be imparting to you to lose those additional loads.

Furthermore, that is the thing you will learn in the accompanying book that I've named, 9 Simple Weight reduction stunts: Lose 10 lbs quick.

I want to believe that you partake in the book.

Take care of You

The greatest propensity that gives you most extreme outcomes for least exertion is the manner by which you deal with your body and what you are placing into your body. On the off chance that you substitute the mentality with which you treat your body for a superior one, getting thinner turns into significantly more straightforward.

You likely definitely realize that a positive routine and a superior routine change to everyday living is one of the least difficult ways of shedding pounds, but no one appears to make it happen; we can't help thinking about why we start to feel as such on the grounds that the vast majority depend on an "go big or go home" approach. With this sort of propensity, they plan to be 100% severe and never surrender to any enticement or oneself loss cycle that could kick in. Nonetheless, what I suggest is that you dissect your dietary propensities and make little replacements that could hugely affect your weight reduction venture. The initial step is to more readily comprehend the food varieties and beverages that you put into your body as well as your day to day daily schedule.

That is the reason, in this segment, we'll zero in on a two dimensional way to deal with settling on more brilliant utilization choices and sound schedules.

In particular, we will discuss the accompanying:

1.	What you drink
2.	What you eat
3.	Your everyday practice

Sounds basic, isn't that so?

To start with, we should discuss perhaps of the greatest guilty party that may be crashing your endeavors at lessening your weight: what you drink.

MIND YOUR Beverages

Various examinations (like this one) have found that drinking bountiful measures of sweet refreshments can build the gamble of putting on weight and creating type 2 diabetes, coronary illness, and gout.

There is a critical relationship between's sweet beverages, weight gain, and stoutness. This is on the grounds that your body isn't intended for drinking calories. You're bringing calories into your body in a manner it isn't expected to manage. For that reason sweet beverage calories are more awful than some other approach to getting calories from sugar.

Ladies who drink at least one sweet refreshments everyday twofold the gamble of creating diabetes contrasted with the people who drink short of what one beverage daily. A youngster's gamble of becoming fat increments by 60% with every day to day sweet beverage they polish off, and the gamble of dental cavities nearly copies in kids who drink carbonated, sweet refreshments.

Sugar drinks are one of the most perilous and tricky ways of slipping calories and synthetic substances into your eating regimen. Sugar drinks are omnipresent, and they're so firmly connected with specific occasions that we polish off them automatically. At the point when outsiders visit America, they're frequently stunned at the size of the soda pops they get when they go to a drive-through joint or the films.

There are general stores where you can get a 64-ounce soda directly from the wellspring machine. Ponder how much sugar is in there. A can is horrible enough for you, however as a general public, we've become OK with drinking from one of these monster cups of pop.

As a matter of fact, a few places much proposition a rebate if you have any desire to go from little to extra-huge. The investment funds are influential for such an extent that it turns out to be practically overpowering. At the point when you have the

The choice to either purchase water or a soda at a similar cost appears to be practically counter-intuitive. At any rate, it resembles you're squandering cash purchasing water when water ought to be free.

Tragically, sweet beverages are obtrusive in our general public. Almost 50% of the U.S. populace drinks somewhere around one sweet beverage each and every day, and five percent drink at least four soft drinks consistently.

In the event that you're attempting to get thinner, wiping out soft drink from your eating regimen is an extraordinary spot to begin. Only one daily will eliminate a critical number of calories. Furthermore, don't be tricked by the name "diet pop." These are not really great for your eating routine. Counterfeit sugars influence your digestion such that triggers weight gain.

Water Is the Response!

So what would it be a good idea for you to drink over the course of the day? The least complex and best choice is to methodicallly supplant the beverages you have with regular water (or water with a tad of lemon or lime in it). There are an assortment of medical advantages of drinking water over the course of the day:
1.   Water works on regularphysical processes.

Getting the right equilibrium of supplements for your body relies upon drinking sufficient water. There is 60% water in your body. Your body cycles can run all the more easily when you're hydrated. You really want water in your body to ship supplements, keep up with your internal heat level, digest and assimilate food, and course blood. Water is the main component in your body since you are for the most part water.

2.   Water stimulates your muscles.

Muscle cells won't work well when they need more liquid. The deficiency of electrolytes and liquids is brought about by muscle exhaustion. To supplant the liquids you lose during exercise, you ought to polish off water. As per American School of Sports Medication rules, 17 minutes is a lot of chance to work out

During any demanding games movement, drink eight extra ounces of water. Exercise ought to be done early and frequently to receive the rewards. Stay away from drying out brought about by perspiring by drinking water before it is required.

3.   Water eliminates poisons. Water eliminates poisons.

Perfect and unadulterated water works really hard of flushing out poisons from the body through sweat, defecations, and pee.

4.   Water expands your energy levels.

A body starts to show thirst at around one to two percent parchedness. As per studies, even before you start to feel parched, the impacts of gentle lack of hydration can diminish energy, mind-set, and thinking. The more dried out a body gets, the lower the energy levels will be.

5.   Water reinforces the invulnerable framework.

Water is a key to wellbeing. Parchedness compromises the body's invulnerable framework. There are many insusceptible framework benefits from appropriate hydration. Water:
*   Oxygenates the blood
*   Eliminates poisons from the blood
*   Increments lymph creation
*   Cleans eyes
*   Cleans mouth
*   Helps digest food
*   Helps battle sleep deprivation
*   Greases up joints
*   Increments serotonin creation (battles gloom)

As may be obvious, besides the fact that water assists with weight reduction, a remedy gives various medical advantages. Things being what they are, how much water would it be a good idea for you to drink?

Indeed, the guideline for the perfect proportion of water admission is eight 8 ounce glasses each day (or a sum of 64 ounces). This number will change as indicated by your weight and level of actual work. As a matter of fact, I will encourage you to get the container that has fine times on it so you can stay aware of your day to day objective and keep focused with the times.

To keep it basic, I suggest purchasing a 32-ounce water bottle, topping it off first thing, and drinking the entire thing.

It is even prudent that you take a glass of water before every dinner. Doing this, you'll see your segments get more modest, your yearning decreases, and the remainder of this interaction turns into significantly simpler.

At last, your objective ought to be to eat calories and not drink them in the event that you would be able, hydrate. Make it somewhat more delightful by blending it in with lemon or different natural products, cucumber, or spices and flavors; that is completely fine. Yet, we need to pursue where sweet beverages never again lose your size of sweet.

WATCH WHAT YOU EAT

The second piece of this propensity is to settle on more intelligent food choices. In particular, The eating routine ought to incorporate every one of the fundamental supplements like sugars, proteins, nutrients, fats, minerals, and water in the suitable extents. This diet is known as a reasonable eating regimen, as it comprises of various fundamental supplements that influence the development and improvement of a body. A totally adjusted diet contributes towards adjusting the supplements that add to keeping up with

Great wellbeing and the executives of weight. Eating a reasonable eating routine will assist you with shedding a couple of pounds without putting you on a prohibitive eating routine.

At the point when you begin following a decent eating regimen, your body gets great sustenance, aside from aiding you in diminishing your weight and furthermore keeping you healthy. You must comprehend what might be a solid eating routine and how much amount of food you can devour each day, which can keep you from being impacted by unfriendly medical issue like hypertension, coronary illness, being overweight, and so on since every one of these are avoidable ailments, if we can stringently follow a restrained way of life by consolidating the right eating regimen for our body followed by a couple of activities to remain solid and fit generally.

Benefits Got from Following A Reasonable Eating regimen:

There are a lot of advantages that you get from following a legitimate and adjusted diet. You can lose overabundance weight, as well as significantly restricting the possibilities being impacted by ongoing as well as non-transmittable illnesses. We should recollect that by following a less than stellar eating routine, we could likewise risk being impacted by specific kinds of malignant growth. This multitude of illnesses have made great many individuals from across the globe be impacted harshly, aside from an ascent in the quantity of passings that has been seen all around the world in the beyond couple of many years, which is an immediate outcome of an undesirable way of life followed by people.
As we have seen before above, you actually should consume the fundamental supplements that are referenced beneath through dietary sources, which can assist you with remaining sound.

Utilization of Nutrients and Minerals for your body:

We as a whole require a lot of nutrients and minerals for our bodies consistently. On the off chance that an individual is encountering an inadequacy or absence of nutrients and minerals that are expected for the individual's body, it might prompt the individual being impacted by any type of weakness.

Numerous people actually are not totally mindful or experience the ill effects of an absence of information on the significance of nutrients and minerals that ought to be incorporated as a feature of their eating routine. An immense number of people have a lack of nutrients and minerals in their bodies. Hence, it is constantly recommended that people incorporate new vegetables like yams, carrots, spinach, and other dull salad greens into their eating regimen.
Also, new natural products, for example, kiwi natural product or citrus natural products like oranges, grapes, and so on, can be consumed by people to shield themselves from any lack in such nutrients and minerals. Further, including specific sorts of dairy items and different grains into their diet is suggested.
Nutrients can do ponders for your body. For example, by devouring food varieties plentiful in nutrients C and E, you are working on your capacity to battle sicknesses, aside from working on your body's resistance.

Likewise, you require food sources that are plentiful in different kinds of nutrients, for example, Vitamin A (helps your vision), Vitamin D (keeps your bones solid), and a couple of others.
Essentially, your body likewise expects minerals to keep up with great wellbeing. For example, calcium is one of the significant minerals that assistance in the arrangement of your teeth as well as bones. Different minerals, for example, iron and magnesium are fundamental for your body, and food varieties containing these parts should be incorporated as a piece of your eating routine.
Iron is a significant mineral that aides in blood arrangement, particularly red platelets called hemoglobin, which really moves the oxygen from the lungs to the wide range of various pieces of the body. Also, supplements, for example, magnesium are expected for your body, as it performs numerous exercises, like controlling the elements of your nerves and muscles. Aside from that, it assists in the guideline of blood with sugaring levels in people and furthermore helps in the avoidance of the event of constant illnesses like sort 2 diabetes, including other cardiovascular sicknesses. Furthermore, it might likewise give help to people from headache or even forestall the event of headache.

Utilization of Sugars and Proteins for your body:

Starches are required for the body of each and every person in great sums consistently. Since you infer sufficient necessary energy for playing out your everyday exercises, you can't easily overlook consuming them. A few wellsprings of sugars like rice, wheat, potatoes, and bread should be consumed by you in adequate amounts with the goal that you would have the option to keep up with the necessary energy for your body. The people who are taken part in active work would require more starches in their eating routine.

Essentially, proteins go about as muscle heads and are important for people to accomplish nice development and improvement of their bodies. In addition, developing children would require a decent level of protein to be integrated into their eating routine.
Proteins assume a critical part in keeping your bones and muscles solid. A protein-rich eating routine is useful for you to acquire elevated degrees of energy, aside from having the option to assist you with shedding pounds. You can begin taking dairy items with low-fat substance, like milk, yogurt, and cheddar, aside from taking eggs, lentils, fish, nuts, kidney beans, and a couple of more to fill your energy necessities consistently. The people who are in the field of sports and different exercises that require high energy levels are expected to make an eating regimen that is wealthy in protein obligatory.

In this way, it is profoundly fundamental for you to follow a decent eating routine by adding suitable amounts of the relative multitude of fundamental supplements as a component of your eating routine consistently to lose overabundance weight and stay solid.

Oversee Feelings of anxiety AND Rest soundly

The third piece of this propensity is to have a legitimate pressure the executives strategy. We've all known about the survival reaction. The capacity to take off from or ward off a saber-toothed tiger is something to be thankful for. The issue with present day stressors is they frequently aren't resolvable through battling or escaping. Things could be such a ton simpler if you would smack your manager upside the head and take off from that very distressing Monday early daytime meeting, couldn't they?

All things considered, the majority of our pressure comes from circumstances we can only with significant effort address. A high-pressure work, contending family commitments, and cash inconveniences are complicated circumstances requiring complex goals that aren't really served by a survival reaction. Tragically, these are probably the most widely recognized types of cutting edge pressure, and accordingly, our pressure reaction is abused.

The Cortisol Reaction

While encountering 'typical' stressors or dangers to your own wellbeing, similar to a major canine jumping at you, the body's pressure reaction framework is self-restricting, implying that once the apparent danger has passed, chemical levels get back to business as usual. However, when stressors are generally present, such is the situation with most current pressure, that survival response stays turned on.

At the point when focused, the body delivers a mixed drink of chemicals intended to help you in tending to and mitigating the stressor. One of these chemicals is called cortisol, and when constantly raised, cortisol can genuinely affect your capacity to get thinner.

This is the carefully guarded secret:

One of cortisol's principal capabilities is to supply the body with energy during a time of pressure to satisfy the physiological needs put on it. Cortisol gives this energy by making glucose through a cycle called gluconeogenesis, a metabolic series happening in the liver where put away protein is changed over into glucose. This rush of glucose energy is intended to help a singular battle or escape the stressor.

Long haul pressure brings about the nonstop creation of glucose, making drawn out, raised glucose levels. At the point when glucose levels are raised, our pancreas is compelled to deliver gigantic measures of insulin to get glucose levels once again to ordinary. Within the sight of this much insulin, our cells become safe, and we can't consume fat. Consider insulin the "guard" that permits or confines

Admittance to our fat stores. Low degrees of insulin permit our cells to deliver fat-put away energy, while elevated degrees of insulin trigger our bodies to clutch it.

Compounding an already painful situation, reliably high blood glucose levels, alongside insulin obstruction, persuades our cells to think they are starving. Those phones are shouting out for energy, and one method for managing that is to convey hunger messages to the cerebrum. This can prompt gorging and deep desires for weighty glucose food sources (carbs), which just intensify the cycle. Furthermore, obviously, all the unusable glucose you've been set off to eat is at last put away as more muscle versus fat.

Step by step instructions to Battle Pressure

Now that we comprehend what stress and cortisol adversely mean for your

weight reduction endeavors, here are a few things you can do about it.

The body is astounding in that it has underlying controllers intended to check itself when a reaction like "an excess of cortisol" is available. Figuring out how to normally actuate or expand the presence of these controllers is critical to assisting you with capitalizing on your weight reduction endeavors.

Development chemical is a restricting cortisol chemical, significance expanded degrees of development chemical stifle the degree of cortisol in your body. It is enacted through rest, exercise, and low blood glucose levels. The last one is precarious on the grounds that we definitely realize cortisol raises blood glucose levels. We'll get to that in a moment, yet we should begin with the initial two.

Rest

I'll concede I'm not an excellent sleeper. I love to rest once I arrive, however I oppose hitting the sack and normally wind up remaining up past the point of no return. I'm on my telephone way as well

Much, thinking excessively, attempting to press another exchange the securities exchange, or I feel anxious and can't settle in.

At the point when we're worn out, we settle on unfortunate choices. What's more, frequently, perhaps of the most unfortunate choice we can make is to enjoy voraciously consuming food or potentially late-evening stacking. Thus, a straightforward weight reduction procedure is to get an entire night's rest reliably.

To get more rest or to work on the nature of your rest, attempt the accompanying:

Keep a steady rest wake cycle: Get up and Save a similar time for nodding off each evening (even on ends of the week). By doing this, you will improve the nature of your rest and set your body's inside clock. Your body ought to consequently awaken without an alert while you're getting sufficient rest. Morning timers can be useful if necessary; it could be an indication that you want a previous sleep time.

Be brilliant about resting: I effectively get found out in the rest cycle by nodding off at night, snoozing for a really long time, and afterward not having the option to nod off at sleep time. Compensating for rest misfortune is conceivable by snoozing; it makes falling or staying unconscious around evening time troublesome. In the event that you should have a rest, restrict it to 15-20 minutes and just in the afternoon at the extremely most recent.

Stay away from splendid screens inside 1-2 hours of sleep time: There are various investigations cautioning us that sleep time screen utilization is one of the main sources of unfortunate rest quality. In the event that you're a telephone crummy like me, take a stab at establishing a point in time when your telephone goes down, and you don't pick it back up again until morning. On the off chance that you're not exactly prepared to bring an end to the propensity for evening telephone use, at least, plan your telephone to switch over to an evening setting to obstruct the blue light that slows down melatonin creation.

Practice care

A condition of care includes being right now with mindfulness and nonjudgment. Contemplation and yoga frequently integrate care strategies. Stress can be decreased through care, a method that has been demonstrated compelling.

The program further develops flexibility, increments mindfulness, diminishes nervousness and wretchedness, and further develops adapting capacity to constant agony. Veterans can work on their lives by rehearsing care consistently, as it can revamp the cerebrum as fast as about two months. There are a few medical advantages related with yoga:

- Further develops mind-set - Uneasiness, and gloom might be diminished with care preparing. The viability of care preparing in forestalling sadness backslide was equivalent to that of antidepressants, as per a review.

- Decreases pressure and its ramifications - The act of care can lessen the force of pressure responses. Pulse is brought down, and your resistant framework is reinforced by doing this.

- Further develops adapting to torment - Care contemplation lessens agony and trouble connected with persistent agony in individuals with constant torment. Their aggravation doesn't keep them from being dynamic.

- Further develops cerebrum capabilities - You can work on your concentration and consideration by rehearsing care. Memory and mental execution can be worked on through this preparation after some time.

- Assists with weight the executives - Stoutness and gorging can be diminished through care methods.

What Are Some Normal Care Strategies?

We have illustrated a couple of care practices here in short. There are a considerable lot of these activities you can do anyplace, even in a hurry, on the off chance that you have some tranquil time. Look at the Assets segment for more data on these strategies.

- Careful breathing - Contemplation can be all around as straightforward as breathing carefully. Center around how your contemplations and breath move in and out as you center your mindfulness without endeavoring to alter them.

- Body check - Notice any actual sensations you feel, sitting or resting, without responding or passing judgment on them. Beginning with the bottoms of the feet, a body sweep could likewise incorporate a look at the knees, hips, back, midsection, chest, and neck.

- Careful eating - Gradually and intentionally biting and gulping your food while focusing on the vibes that happen as you hold, smell, taste, bite, and swallow it.

- Adoring generosity contemplation - Righteous reasoning and wish-allowing is an activity that includes zeroing in first on yourself, then, at that point, on your dearest companions and family, then on additional far off colleagues, and afterward on every other person in the world.

- Careful development - Be aware of your breathing, your body developments, and the general climate while strolling or rolling. Zeroing in on your actual sensations while breathing in and breathing out each posture is one more method for rehearsing care.

Eat soundly

This next one is somewhat trickier. As referenced before, having low blood glucose levels Lifts your body's creation of development chemicals. Amazing! But we definitely realize that elevated degrees of cortisol increment blood glucose levels — so what else is there to do?

Most importantly, following a decent eating routine is an extraordinary method for decreasing and deal with your general blood glucose levels. Assuming you're as of now doing that, continue onward! Assuming that you suspect that ongoing elevated degrees of cortisol are as yet hindering your weight reduction endeavors (as they've done I would say), you might need to integrate a smidgen of discontinuous fasting into your fair eating routine. This might mean giving yourself a deadline when you quit eating for the night, postponing your most memorable feast of the day, or both.

At the point when in an abstained state (like first thing), your body delivers the Insulin-Like Development Variable. IGF is a controller chemical, like development chemical, in that it brings down cortisol. While insulin is answerable for controlling glucose levels while eating, insulin-like development factor manages glucose levels while you're not eating. Whenever you allow yourself an opportunity to not eat, you're consequently diminishing your blood glucose levels while likewise delivering cortisol inhibitors like development chemical and insulin-like development factors.

HAVE A Sound WEIGHING Schedule

Another thing I will include this segment is a matter that has turned into an object of discussion. It is tied in with gauging yourself and keeping tabs on your development.

Indeed, it is likewise an approach to dealing with yourself, yet to remain sound, there's nobody estimation that fits all. Scales get a terrible standing since individuals depend entirely on them.

It can in any case be trying to gauge yourself. Is there a specific scale you ought to get? While building muscle, would it be advisable for you to gauge yourself? With regards to simply getting in shape, is it unique?

If I somehow managed to gauge myself accurately, how might I make it happen?

Gauge yourself...

- 1x week

- in the mornings

- same way like clockwork (e.g., in the wake of crapping, regardless of garments)

- with a tracker

- Provided that it doesn't set off uneasiness or confused eating

1. Weigh yourself one time each week

It's enticing to bounce on the scale consistently in the event that you're keeping tabs on your development

Try not to make it happen.

"Gauging yourself more frequently than once seven days isn't needed. Rachel Fine, the proprietor of To The Pointe Nourishment and enrolled dietitian, says everyday water variances can definitely change body weight.

" It will be simpler for you to monitor your weight by gauging yourself the same way consistently."

2. Weigh yourself toward the beginning of the day

Subsequent to drinking water or eating a dinner, don't step aerobics the scale just after you gauge yourself. At the point when you gauge yourself promptly in the first part of the day, you will come by the most reliable outcomes.

"Gauging yourself first thing works best on the grounds that your stomach related framework has had sufficient opportunity to process and process your food (you had a short-term quick). An enrolled dietitian at Nutri Sharp Wellbeing, Lauren O'Connor, says eating or handling won't influence it."

3. Keep elements predictable

Downplay the factors on the scale assuming you maintain that the number should be precise. Weight changes will not entirely set in stone by whether you are exposed or in exercise garments - still up in the air by how much weight you have acquired or lost every week. (Shoes don't count!)

Consistency is significant with regards to gauging yourself. You ought to likewise gauge yourself at the same time. The following time you bounce onto the scale, go to the washroom first.

Weighingyourselfwithoutclothes?Keepitthatway,ortrywearingthesameclothes weektoweek.

4. Track your advancement

A week after week weight check is important for your daily practice. On the scale, you see a diminishing in weight. Monitoring your advancement will truly assist you boost your relationship with your scale.

You'll have the option to distinguish designs, have a superior feeling of how things are going, and be persuaded to remain focused to arrive at your weight reduction objectives, in any event, when you need to surrender.

Could it be better in the event that it were programmed? Consider putting resources into a savvy scale that you can interface with your telephone by means of an application. Also, shrewd scales measure something other than weight, including muscle to fat ratio and bulk, to more readily grasp your general wellbeing.

5. Completely trench the scale

Surrendering the scale is alright, especially on the off chance that it's not working on your wellbeing or confidence.
Did it give you nervousness when you attempted it? Try not to burn through your time.
Its presence triggers negative considerations, does it not? Put it in the rubbish and think of it as a weight reduction of 2 pounds! You might find that you could do without the scale, yet progress is much of the time the best estimation.
In the event that you experience the ill effects of a dietary issue or have disarranged dietary patterns, having a scale in your home may not be fundamental. Weight-ins can be passed on to your medical care supplier so you can focus on different things that make you cheerful and solid.

Dealing with yourself is a vital piece of the stunt. This is on the grounds that when you are looking great and your mentality is right, shedding pounds turns out to be simple.

Now that we've dealt with you, how about we move to the following stunt!

MOVE YOUR BODY

People tend to look at wellness experts and expect they are consistently in the mood to train, or that all they do is to get into the exercise center or work out their wellness through sorts of hardware. You actually should comprehend this doesn't need to take serious power lifting or hours on the treadmill for you to work out. It's vital to comprehend that any development is a type of activity.

Fundamental Developments ARE ALL THAT'S Required

I suggest that you search for amazing open doors over the course of the day to increment and integrate greater development into your day. A few models may be doing squats as you clean your teeth, running to the letter box and around the block before you return home, more squats while doing the dishes, strolling a portion of a mile to the corner shop as opposed to driving, or continuously using the stairwell (rather than the lift) in structures. You can likewise incorporate key extending occasionally all through your normal business day, using the stairwell to the workplace, stopping in the farthest spot from the entryway when you make your staple run, or doing bouncing jacks during ads as you watch your number one show. I'll be quick to concede that these thoughts sound perfect in principle yet can be difficult to integrate into a bustling timetable. I have framed three moves toward further guarantee that you amplify each development that you get.

Step #1: Wear a Stage GPS beacon

A stage tracker is just a little gadget or a watch that tracks the number of steps you that require over the course of the day and the number of floors you that trip. Essentially following the number of steps you that require over the course of the day can incredibly affect your actual wellness.

At the point when you get to work, you likely take the lift. Yet, in the event that you have a stage tracker with you, you'll understand you get more "focuses" for going up the steps, and the chances of you going up those steps increment. You're bound to stop farther away in the

Parking area since now you're getting credit for it. The most horrendously awful thing about practicing is when no one notification your endeavors. In the event that you get no credit, it feels futile. Step counters guarantee that you get the credit you merit.

From the outset, it could appear to be that putting on a stage GPS beacon is an immaterial step, yet that is on the grounds that individuals purchase these gadgets and never connect them to their bodies. Your morning schedule ought to continuously incorporate cut-out this gadget to your body, and that is the initial step to building an activity propensity.

Step #2: Walk 250 to 500 Stages Consistently

The best and most straightforward method for practicing is to walkways to get normal activity without adversely affecting your bustling timetable. While it's essential to have a standard work-out daily schedule (which we'll discuss in the following subtopic), you can work on your endeavors on the off chance that you simply walk an extra 250 to 500 stages consistently. This joins two positive propensities.

In the first place, it battles against every one of the unfortunate results of sitting a lot over the course of the day; and second, strolling for two to five minutes consistently gives a fast mental break from your work. The vast majority normal 100 stages of strolling each moment. That implies strolling five minutes will get you 500 stages. Assuming you focus on enjoying one of these reprieves multiple times every day, that is 5,000 stages, which is most of the way to that 10,000-step objective that a great many people have when they wear stride trackers.

Step #3: Augment Little Pockets of Time

In the event that you're a bustling individual who's consistently in a hurry and essentially can't carve out opportunity to finish a work-out daily schedule at the rec center DVD exercise, then, at that point, this is the ideal procedure for you. You want to expand your development by boosting each little bit of time you have over the course of the day. That is the reason I suggest step trackers: Each step counts. Furthermore, you can expand these means by adding little pieces of development over the course of the day. Here is a rundown of thoughts you can carry out:

• You can pace while sitting tight for a gathering of any sort, whether you are at a physical checkup, holding up in line at the Branch of Engine Vehicles, or getting your children after school. Regardless of whether you simply pace for a few minutes, you'll have 240 to 360 stages in a few minutes at 120 stages each moment.

• While you're shopping, stroll along the farthest walkways in the event that you're in no hurry. As well as checking for specials you might have missed the initial time, you can stroll all over each path once more in the event that you like.

• Utilize the bathroom on the following floor, up or down, instead of the nearest one at work. Use the stairwell rather than the lift.

- Advance toward the television or Cd player to change the station. As opposed to utilizing the remote, change the music player on your PC physically. Instead of depending on a mechanized framework, stroll around the house. Assuming you like to do your dishes by hand instead of utilizing the dishwasher, mark the time. Make your home an imaginative spot.
- You ought to stroll around the house as opposed to plunking down and chatting on the telephone.
- Make your collaborators part of the interaction. You can have a gathering outside while strolling whenever there's a gathering.
- In the event that it doesn't cause you excessive deferral, keep away from lifts and lifts.
- Going for a heartfelt stroll after supper will assist you with consuming off calories on the off chance that you are seeing someone.
- Watch the dawn or nightfall from a beautiful area promptly toward the beginning of the day. Rather than going out for supper, consolidate this thought with the final remaining one and plan a cookout.
- Go for a stroll after chapel as opposed to going to the espresso hour in the event that you go to chapel.

By zeroing in on non-weight-related As opposed to fear moving, you can energize sensations of bliss encompassing it.

1. Enhanced State of mind

The demonstration of moving your body isn't just helpful for your temperament, however it is additionally compelling for engaging sadness and nervousness. The information demonstrate that exercise can give these advantages to people of any age and genders, paying little mind to mental problems.

Stress can likewise be adapted to through work out. Specialists requested that members play out an unpleasant undertaking and a non-distressing control task in a review. A critical decrease in good effect (mind-set) was accounted for by the people who didn't practice no less than once seven days subsequent to following through with the distressing responsibility, as well as feeling unpleasant for the most part. As well as keeping a positive state of mind and keeping pressure from collecting in your body, routine work-out may likewise keep you from encountering intense pressure.

2. Healthier Lymph

In your body, lymphatics are a piece of the resistant framework. The main thing you are familiar lymph hubs is in the event that your throat is sore and you feel a knot in your neck. All through the body, the lymph framework is made out of hubs and channels which move lymph liquid. There are white platelets in the lymph liquid that are answerable for battling disease all through the body. Eliminating possibly unsafe poisons and microscopic organisms from the body assumes a critical part in the resistant framework.

The lymphatic framework utilizes your movement to circle lymph liquid rather than a siphon, similar to the circulatory or respiratory frameworks. Lymphatic liquid courses through your body when you move huge muscles of the body.

3. Healthier Bones

Muscles are not by any means the only thing that can be profited from work out. It is additionally gainful to keep up with and construct bone mass when you move back and forth against your bones. Building bone mass is best achieved through weight-bearing activities. You don't need to utilize loads to achieve this. You can construct bone mass by strolling, moving, or using the stairwell for a supported timeframe. Bone development is bound to happen with higher effects.

Practice is significant for building bones all through your life. The most ideal way to make thick bones for kids is to participate in customary active work since youngsters keep on building bones until about almost 90% of the bone mass in an individual's body is gathered when they arrive at the age of 20.

It is normal for bone mass to decline after the age of thirty. Cracks are normal among the older as a result of solid problems like osteoporosis. You can keep up with bone mass by working out, despite the fact that some level of bone misfortune can't be kept away from.

1. **Enhanced Brain Health**

People of all ages benefit from exercise when it comes to cognitive performance. Researchers found that children participating in physical activity showed improved mental accuracy and reaction times as well as increased electrical activity in their brains. An additional study confirmed what was intuitive obvious-that a healthy exercise routine in childhood may contribute to your cognitive decline later in life.

42 years later, physical activity was less likely to be associated with early-onset dementia and mild cognitive impairment in individuals who were physically active at 18 years of age.

2. Improved Sex Life

Both men and women benefit from exercise in terms of their sex lives (arousal and satisfaction). As well as improving sexual function for men, regular exercise may contribute to feeling "in the mood" by improving psychosocial factors like mood, stress, and confidence. In addition, by building muscle mass, interval cardio workouts and weightlifting may increase testosterone levels as well.

Surrendering the scale is alright, especially in the event that it's not working on your wellbeing or confidence.

Did it give you uneasiness when you attempted it? Try not to burn through your time.

Its presence triggers negative considerations, does it not? Put it in the rubbish and think of it as a weight reduction of 2 pounds! You might find that you could do without the scale, yet progress is many times the best estimation.

On the off chance that you experience the ill effects of a dietary problem or have scattered dietary patterns, having a scale in your home may not be vital. Weight-ins can be passed on to your medical services supplier so you can focus on different things that make you blissful and sound.

Dealing with yourself is a vital piece of the stunt. This is on the grounds that when you are looking great and your disposition is right, getting thinner turns out to be simple.

Now that we've dealt with you, how about we move to the following stunt!

What Kind of Activity?

Instead of give you a particular and nitty gritty activity system, it's better for you to fit one to your body and current condition. Your activity routine ought to be worked around your ongoing degree of actual capacity, as well as your movement, actual capability, wellbeing, practice reactions, expressed objectives, and how much leisure time that you have accessible to devote to work out. On the off chance that you need more opportunity to hit a 30-minute exercise five days per week, it's actually better to practice for five minutes every morning than to not do anything by any stretch of the imagination. Adding activity to your routine decreases how much time you spend taking a seat at work. A little activity during noon can fundamentally affect your day.

The main piece of your activity routine is that it should be something you appreciate. On the off chance that you disdain yoga, going to yoga five days seven days won't work since you'll be in a steady condition of contention, accomplishing something you disdain as opposed to something you appreciate. The excellence is that exercise is surrounding you. Anyplace on the planet you live, there are hundreds and even a huge number of activity choices for you to browse. On the off chance that you're now executing the technique from the past area and getting development over the course of the day, adding this next layer will make you relentless. Also, on the off chance that you're hitting your day to day development and step objectives, I recommend you start with a work-out routine where you're turning out for 30 to 45 minutes something like four times each week. The following inquiry, obviously, kind of activity routine you ought to follow.

Step #1: Pick practice programs that you're keen on.

Practice doesn't need to exhaust! We as a whole have individual inclinations about which sports exercises we appreciate and hate. I have consistently delighted in moving, strolling,

furthermore, different sorts of fun exercises, while many individuals believe it's a type of relaxation. That is the very thing that I appreciate, yet what you lean toward may be unique. That is the reason I don't suggest a specific activity as a definitive exercise to do. I feel that a choice ought to be made in light of your circumstance and how long you can dedicate to work out. All things considered, with regards to shedding pounds, it has been exhibited that coming up next are the best kinds of exercises for consuming calories:

- Swimming
- Strength preparing
- Running
- Strolling

- CrossFit
- Extreme cardio exercise.
- Body weight works out (hopping jacks, pushups, burpees, hikers, and so on.)
- Yoga
- Working out with rope
- Step climbing machines (or just strolling up a bumpy course)
- Cycling span preparing (i.e., a quick moving twist class)
- Kickboxing

These are only a modest bunch of thoughts you could integrate into your timetable. However, on the off chance that you can't choose the "great" work out, then, at that point, I ask you to have a go at something. As I said previously, any kind of development is not all that great, but not terrible either than nothing, so don't allow uncertainty to keep you from making a move. Simply pick a couple of choices and bounce in.

Step #2: Teach yourself on the nuts and bolts.

You don't have to have a deep understanding of an activity to make a plunge — you simply have to know to the point of beginning. There are countless recordings, webcasts, and books about working out. You basically have to recognize a couple of connected with your movement of interest and do a little research. You don't need to take an excess of time with your exploration. Simply search for a fast fledgling's aide that assists you with getting everything rolling without gambling with injury.

Step #3: Talk with a specialist in advance.

Before we continue on, I exceptionally propose you converse with your primary care physician and see what they suggest for your age and actual capacity. Make certain to get a total physical. Additionally, discuss your own clinical history, your family clinical history, any previous issues you had with working out, any previous wounds, any sort of activity you might want to attempt, and, obviously, any different kinds of feedback you have about this activity.

Step #4: Practice structure and procedure.

Before you fabricate an exercise around a particular action, learning the correct method for doing it is significant. That is the reason I suggest putting in a couple of days in purposeful practice.

Step #5: Timetable activity into your day.

There might be times when life conditions keep you from practicing according to plan. You know the situation — you planned to work out, yet something sprung up that removed time from it. You have work interruptions or the "only another email" issue. You continue to intend to begin on your miniature responsibility, yet you need to answer that message, Skype message, email, and so forth. It never appears to end. In all actuality you will constantly have interferences. In the event that you let these interferences direct your life, you will never at any point achieve anything past the prompt needs of your work and individual life. This is called endurance mode — extinguishing many flames as they spring up. This is horrible quality of life, and it unquestionably isn't a method for flourishing and benefit from life.

What I prescribe is to utilize the in the event that arranging idea to distinguish potential activity deterrents before they occur. Begin every day by booking when you'll exercise, and afterward distinguish each conceivable thing that could intrude on this action. Then, at that point, make a progression of plans for how you'll deal with the interferences if/when they come your direction.
Step #6: Track your exercises.

Rivaling others and following your wellness propensities are incredible ways of propelling yourself. Frequently, this can give that additional push when you don't feel available. An extraordinary method for doing this is with applications and wearable gadgets that screen your action.

Step #7: Keep at it!

From the beginning, adding activity to your day will feel like a test. There will be days when you'll feel unmotivated — however keep at it! Before long, feeling totally normal to you is going. Your body was intended to move around the entire day, not to sit in an office or on a lounge chair for significant length of time. Your body is very much like anything more — on the off chance that you don't involve it for its planned reason, it begins to fizzle. Figuring out how to bring exercise into your life will go quite far toward broadening your life by many years.

The significance of activity is it works on your body and keeps you better. It battles illness and assists you with living longer. It helps you have an improved outlook on yourself and holds you back from gaining weight. The advantages of activity for our wellbeing are notable. Be that as it may, assuming you search in the mirror and say, "I realize practice is great for me, for what reason don't I don't make it happen?" the response is frequently, "I need more time" or "I hate it any longer." We need to find exercises you appreciate since, supposing that practicing is a joy, you're bound to do it than if it's a task. That is the reason I'll urge you to find exercises that are pleasurable and tomfoolery and that require a smidgen of development. Assuming there's a movement that hits each and every one of your activity objectives, however you disdain getting it done, and one more action that hits 80% of your objectives and you love making it happen, seek after action number two. Enthusiasm and want will assist you with overcoming the challenge.

PORTION YOUR FOOD

There are things in your home you presumably don't you dare even consider that are neutralizing your eating regimen. A plate's size is something you ought to consider. Food choice and part control are similarly significant when you need to get more fit or keep a solid weight.

It is normal to mistake segment sizes for serving sizes, however there is really a contrast between the two. You eat a piece when you eat something at a time. Food serving sizes are the suggested measures of explicit food varieties. At the point when you eat three ounces of chicken for supper, that is a serving, not a piece. Segment control is more straightforward when it are controlled to serve sizes.

We have a thought of how large a plate ought to be for the fundamental course, a canapé, and dessert. However, those sizes are off-base. The typical American eats a few times the suggested serving size of their dinners. At the point when you have a huge plate, it fools you into thinking you want to fill it.

The typical plate size during the 1980s was a little nine-inch plate. Today the normal plate size is 12 inches. The typical cut of pizza? 30% bigger. Normal bagel size? 50% bigger. The rundown continues forever. The fact is that as a populace, we're suffocating in the pile of food that is served in cafés and at home. It feels unnatural to fill a third or even 50% of the plate as it were. Despite the fact that it's an overabundance, and despite the fact that we feel full, we harm ourselves by utilizing larger than average plates. Since you would rather not have an unfilled looking plate, you top it off. Then, at that point, since you feel strain to clean your plate and not appear to be unappreciative of your dinner, you keep eating, even after you feel full.

WHAT ARE THE Advantages OF Part CONTROL?

1. Better assimilation: It is normal for acid reflux and inconvenience to happen when piece sizes are excessively huge. On the off chance that you don't over-burden your stomach related framework with food, it will work better. At the point when bits are made due, cramps and swelling can be stayed away from.

2. Balanced glucose: By over-burdening the body with glucose, indulging can cause glucose irregular characteristics, which can prompt insulin obstruction. Keeping a sound body requires more modest feasts.

3. Improved satiety: A lot of food can prompt a sensation of being full, yet it can likewise prompt not seeing your stomach's signals when it is full. Lessen food utilization by dialing back and seeing yearning prompts.

4. Weight misfortune: Weight reduction can be accomplished by eating more modest parts. You can cut calories and shed undesirable pounds by eating offset feasts with the legitimate serving sizes. Monitoring your weight progress is simple with our Accuracy Tracker Computerized Restroom Scale. At the point when the Tracker is first arranged, up to 8 clients' beginning loads will be logged. A weight change from the last weigh-in to the current weigh-in will be shown on the scale on each ensuing weigh-in.

5. Money investment funds: The quantity of everyday food items you want to purchase will diminish when you eat suggested serving sizes. At the point when trail blend or nuts are allotted, they will endure longer than if they were eaten straight out of the bundle.

SO How Might YOU Fight the temptation TO Top Off A Larger than average PLATE?

The initial step is to purchase and utilize more modest plates.

You ought to never eat from the holders or the bundling the food comes in. Whether it's the fanciest of eateries, a microwavable feast, or a cheap food dinner, don't let holder sizes stunt you. In the event that you put it on a plate, you can more readily evaluate how enormous your feast is. Separate your eating area from your food-readiness area. It does you no decent to carry the holders and the plate to your lounge area table and afterward have those compartments directly before your face enticing you.

Set up your food in the kitchen, move it to a plate of a sensible size, and take that plate to the lounge area. This makes a detachment, so you don't have enticing food directly before you. At the point when you're full, you'll quit eating. The magnificence of a more modest plate is that it will fool your brain into accepting there's more food than there really is. This guideline is known as the Delboeuf deception, which says that encompassing something with bunches of void area causes it to seem more modest. You would rather not do that.

All things considered, utilize a more modest plate so you get the contrary impact — your dinner feels bigger. Investigation into this deception has found that with bigger plates, individuals make mistaken appraisals of serving sizes. The bigger the plate, the more modest they think the serving size is, in any event, when it's the very same. An examination was finished at a wellbeing food camp to perceive how this works out at supper time. They gave the campers different-sized bowls, and those with bigger dishes ate 16% more food than those with more modest dishes.

Enormous dinnerware makes us serve and eat more without taking note. Simultaneously, huge dishes and plates persuade us that we've eaten less. It is smart to keep away from buffets, yet assuming you are placed into that particular situation, snatch the more modest plate. Regardless of whether you top off a more modest plate two times, it's generally expected less food than filling the bigger plate once, and you'll feel like you've eaten more.

Moreover, we can boost the impact by adding an interruption toward the finish of each plate. Toward the finish of each plate. There's a period delay between when you wrap up eating, that second when your stomach is full, and when the sign gets to your mind. During that time delay, Despite the fact that your body has sufficient food, your mind doesn't remember it. You're actually getting the yearning signal, so you keep eating even after you complete the process of feeling hungry. The method for defeating this is to delay or hold for 20 minutes after each and every plate. Eat a little plate and stand by 20 minutes. On the off chance that you're as yet eager, return to the kitchen or make one more excursion to the smorgasbord.

In the event that you don't, then, at that point, you'll have opposed gorging. You're turning out to be more in line with what your body needs and needs. Besides, there are various little propensities transforms you can make that can do ponders for your part control endeavors.

Master serving sizes: Part measures have expanded decisively throughout the course of recent many years, as we have talked about. The outcome is that a great many people underrate the size of servings nowadays.
For this reason figuring out how to peruse food marks is so significant. Since you spend more cash on their items the more you eat, makers configuration marks to be challenging to comprehend. Understanding the measurements behind serving sizes is advantageous eventually. Your body will actually want to let know if you have "enough" food by seeing how you feel.

Utilizing the accompanying piece sizes as specific illustrations, you can without much of a stretch envision information:

- Three ounces (meat or fish) = deck of cards
- 1/2 cup is one frozen yogurt scoop
- One cup is the size of a shut clench hand

Nearly everybody thinks they understand what a part size is, and nearly everybody is off-base. Our view of what's viewed as ordinary has been slanted by the super-sized mindset. The piece size of every dinner still up in the air by knowing the amount to eat.

Use segment control plates: As referenced previously, starting around 1980, the normal plate size has expanded from nine creeps to 12 inches. That is an increment of 33%. So a basic arrangement is to switch this pattern and purchase a 33 percent more modest plate. Top it off however much you need, heaping on the veggies and salad. Like that, you'll be full, satisfied, and eating appropriately estimated dinners.

Pack your extras right away: On the off chance that you have extras after supper, pack them away straightaway. After you unload your extras, you can continuously eat them later on the off chance that you're eager. However long you pack away the food after a solitary dinner, you'll lessen the possibility "eating out of comfort."

Transform a solitary dinner out into two feasts: You ought to possibly eat half of your dinner when you go out to eat. The second your server/server brings your feast, ask them for a "to-go box" and store half for another dinner. The "disagreeableness" of café dinners can't regularly be controlled, however you can lessen the calories in any event.

Plan single-serving bundles: The extras from huge dinners ought to be separated into single-serving bundles. You can then effectively get a lunch for school or work that is impeccably partitioned.

Single word of wariness: Don't get carried away. The outcome? "You'll wind up in a never-ending condition of 'starvation mode,' which frequently brings about gorging followed by the ensuing sensations of responsibility, disgrace, or disappointment from not following your eating regimen," makes sense of metabolic preparation master Nathan Trenteseaux, proprietor of Underground Wellness Unrest in Florida.

An equilibrium of calories in and out is fundamental to acquiring, losing, and keeping up with weight. By giving an excessive number of calories all at once, huge bits of food can adversely influence weight. Indulging and devouring a bigger number of calories than needed can likewise be brought about by enormous bits of food. It is feasible to put on weight assuming that you keep on devouring enormous bits of food. Segment control is a vital stunt to cause the body to accept it is sufficiently taking!

IT'S About Products of the soil

Everybody realizes that products of the soil are a fundamental piece of a solid eating regimen, and the US Branch of Farming rules express that we ought to have something like five servings everyday, yet the normal American eats about three servings per day.

With additional conventional techniques like eating leafy foods, you are bound to get in shape rapidly and keep it off. Foods grown from the ground ought to be seen in a solid and reasonable manner if you have any desire to speed up the weight reduction process.

Many individuals make up for their absence of products of the soil consumption by taking enhancements. In any case, research shows that these are no swap for the supplements found in new products of the soil in light of the fact that these supplements cooperate. For instance, eating spinach, which is wealthy in iron, and drinking squeezed orange, which upgrades the retention of iron thanks to the presence of L-ascorbic acid, is helpful for individuals who need more iron or have iron-lack frailty.

Not in the least do leafy foods work on existing sicknesses or conditions, yet they likewise help in forestalling numerous ailments, including strokes and diabetes. One review that traversed 14 years and followed more than 100,000 individuals presumed that an expansion in everyday utilization of products of the soil prompted a lessening in the possibility creating cardiovascular sicknesses.

Kinds OF Natural product and VEGGIE DIETS

Following a foods grown from the ground diet in more ways than one is conceivable. One of the most straightforward ways of adding fiber and nourishment to your eating regimen is to add a few servings of new produce. By the by, some are more severe than others. Products of the soil make up most of certain individuals' eating regimens, with chicken or fish being a little part. Notwithstanding vegetables, certain individuals drink eggs, yogurt, milk, and cheddar rather than meat. Vegetarian slims down expect that you eat just plant-based food varieties, which are the strictest of all products of the soil counts calories. No subsidiaries

Creatures are permitted. It is feasible to shed pounds with any of these eating routine choices, however going veggie lover might be the quickest method for doing it without imperiling your wellbeing.

Sustenance

As well as assisting you with getting in shape, foods grown from the ground give various medical advantages. Apples, bananas, and blackberries contain vitamin E tomato, kiwi, yam, spinach, oranges, kale, lemons, potatoes, grapes, and avocados containing iron (grapes, avocados, peas, carrots). Strawberries, melon, broccoli, asparagus, zinc, corn, lima beans, and squash contain folic corrosive, zinc, and folic corrosive.

A sound stomach related framework is likewise advanced by them. Accordingly, poisons and waste are kept from developing in the body. You will actually want to get more fit while getting the supplements you want by consuming a products of the soil diet. It's smarter to eat new produce than to eat less carbs like that since the best items on earth are not destructive to your body.

Fiber

You can keep your stomach related framework working appropriately by eating leafy foods. Vegetables with green leaves are especially great sources. You additionally feel fulfilled when you eat less when you consume fiber. You will actually want to get thinner all the more really and consume less calories subsequently.

Water

It is likewise essential to take note of that foods grown from the ground contain a great deal of water. Because of the great water content, you will feel more full quicker than with different food sources, which is positively really great for your body and stomach related framework. Your body consumes more put away fat in the event that you feel more full quicker, and you eat less calories in light of the fact that your body consumes put away fat rather than calories consumed from food.

Nibble Choices

Keeping a sound eating routine that incorporates foods grown from the ground is likewise helpful to those attempting to get in shape. The tidbit contains no calories, cholesterol, fat, sodium, or sugar will in any case fulfill your yearning without topping you off. At the point when you eat new produce, you never feel denied while simultaneously decreasing your caloric admission for speedy weight reduction.

THE Significance OF Foods grown from the ground IN THE HUMAN Eating regimen

You Appreciate Better Wellbeing

How do products of the soil help your wellbeing? Low sugar, salt, and fat levels are tracked down in leafy foods, while fiber levels are high. Keeping a solid weight and lessening corpulence can both be accomplished by eating them.

Leafy foods low in carbs can bring down pulse and cholesterol. As well as battling stroke, type 2 diabetes, cardiovascular sickness, hypertension, and malignant growth, the phytochemicals in the plants will assist with supporting resistance.

You can diminish cholesterol, control your glucose, and manage your craving with fiber in leafy foods. Clogging brought about by a hindered stomach related framework is likewise kept away from.

Foods grown from the ground Are a Fabulous Energy Source

The supplements and supplements in leafy foods are stimulating, heavenly, and nutritious. These are extraordinary in light of the fact that they needn't bother with to be cooked and can be eaten whenever. The energy you get is fundamental for carrying on with a furious life consistently. You will be feeling better on the off chance that you have more energy. As well as keeping the load off, low-carb foods grown from the ground give your body sufficient glucose to ideally work.

There Is Such a lot of Assortment

If you somehow managed to compose a rundown of foods grown from the ground, you could scarcely start to expose what's underneath in regards to what is accessible. You have the decision of lasting through the year or occasional foods grown from the ground.
They come in different varieties and surfaces, further adding to their allure. You can consume them crude or cooked, frozen or new, dried or canned. In the event that you need more assortment, squeezing will give you a cool, sustenance pressed drink.
Do you find that you get in the middle between dinners? In the event that indeed, you might turn to unfortunate eating propensities to battle the food cravings. New products of the soil give a fabulous method for eating. They are filling, and you will feel full longer. You can change around the choices because of the assortment. So the following time you even consider going after that chocolate bar, search for a nutritious and tasty natural product or vegetable all things considered.

They Are an Amazing Wellspring of Minerals and Nutrients

Disregard running for supplements; simply increment your day to day take-up of leafy foods.
A portion of the minerals you will get incorporate nutrients A, C, and E, zinc, folic corrosive, phosphorus, and magnesium. On the off chance that you have very little openness to daylight, eating vitamin D products of the soil like mushrooms, spinach, kale, soybeans, and white beans will guarantee you experience the ill effects of no inadequacies.

Leafy foods Are Savvy Dinner Choices

When contrasted with meat and other creature items, leafy foods are less expensive choices. It's as yet conceivable to appreciate them in such countless ways because of the assortment accessible. There are lots of recipes online that you can follow

assuming you are imaginative or great at following headings.
Natural leafy foods can be drawn from your kitchen garden. It is as yet conceivable to develop your own harvests regardless of whether you have adequate room. The developing system can be controlled, and you can set aside cash. Purchasing new spices from the greengrocer will set aside you cash and forestall the utilization of pesticides and herbicides.

Specialists have additionally looked into the relationship among's leafy foods and disease. Not much is authoritative yet, yet proof recommends that specific vegetables, like broccoli, salad greens, and cabbage, may diminish the probability of mouth, stomach, and colorectal tumors in light of the fact that these vegetables don't contain starch.

One more condition that can be forestalled with leafy foods is overweight or heftiness, which can likewise prompt a huge range of hazardous sicknesses. Since they are low in fat and calories and contain heaps of fiber and water, leafy foods can encourage you without expanding your caloric admission by much.

1.   Fruit assists you with feeling more full for longer: Joanna Foley, RD, CLT, remarks that natural product is a magnificent wellspring of nutrients and minerals, including fiber, that might be useful to you feel full over an extensive stretch of time. This might bring about less calories being consumed, assisting you with getting thinner.
Regardless of the way that natural products are completely intended to top you off, they are not all made equivalent. Which food sources do you suggest for topping off between and during feasts to forestall gorging? Avocados are the universally adored among recent college grads. "Avocados are one of the greatest fiber natural products, as well as giving solid fats, which likewise assist with keeping you full," she says, adding that they can be added to smoothies, sandwiches, or even heated as a sound, fulfilling beating.

2.   Fruits with a high flavonoid content might assist you with trying not to pack on pounds.

"Eating organic product high in flavonoids might assist with weight control and cutoff weight gain. A few classes of flavonoids have been displayed to diminish energy consumption, which can help with weight reduction," says Tara Tomaino, RD, Enrolled Dietitian at The Recreation area, Another Jersey-based work-life grounds that offers health and attendant services, from The Connell Organization. Simply look at this exploration. "Strawberries and blueberries are two natural products high in flavonoids that ought to be remembered for a sound eating routine. Add these luxuriously hued berries to your day by fixing oats, cereal, or yogurt with cut strawberries. Frozen berries are extraordinary added to a bowl of Greek yogurt or to an entire grain biscuit blend," she adds.

3.   Fruit further develops insulin awareness.

"Organic product contains fiber, which forestalls your glucose from spiking a lot of subsequent to eating contrasted with food sources without fiber. This further develops insulin responsiveness, which assists you with shedding pounds," says Foley. You can eat berries all alone for a scrumptious and nutritious treat or add them to smoothies, oats, and yogurt, or use them in smoothie recipes. The accompanying states are the best places to pick berries.

4.   Eating natural product can assist with supporting other solid choices you're making.

Really trying to eat natural product consistently will launch a pattern of useful propensities for you. Diana Gariglio-Clelland, RD, the dietitian for Next Extravagance, states, "Rather than essentially settling on solid decisions (like eating organic product), changing your way of life can prompt weight reduction over the long haul." A nutritionist suggests the nine best organic products for weight reduction as probably the best weight reduction natural products.

As a nourishment master with Grapes from California, Toby Amidor is an honor winning nutritionist with a MS, RD, and CDN degree and an individual from FAND; he suggests a couple of frozen grapes rather than that 16 ounces of sorbet after supper since they are low in sugar and are loaded with cell reinforcements and other polyphenols. Supplant soft drink with natural product smoothies, which are the main wellspring of added sugar in the US," she recommends.

2. Fruit advances a sound stomach microbiome.

Stomach microorganisms are really great for you, so we should get them rolling. The variety of stomach microorganisms can be improved by eating organic product, which exploration shows can be gainful to weight reduction, notices Foley. Apples contain prebiotic fiber, which sustains the microbes in your stomach," she makes sense of, adding that cutting apples into servings of mixed greens or oats are extraordinary ways of partaking in the natural product by some other means than eating them entirety.

VEGETABLES AND Weight reduction

1) Vegetables assist with keeping you full for longer. It is simpler to top off vegetables since they have fiber and water than handled carbs that need fiber. You'll remain fulfilled until your next dinner in the event that you join vegetables with protein and sound fats.

2) Vegetables assist with forestalling dunks and spikes in your energy levels. As well as controlling your glucose, vegetables likewise contain fiber. It is far-fetched that you will experience that late-evening energy rut (and desires for sugar) brought about by eating an excessive amount of handled carbs assuming you consume every one of the vegetables you want every day.

3) Vegetables assist you with living longer. Irritation, an issue related with weight, diabetes, coronary illness, and Alzheimer's sickness, can be forestalled through an eating regimen wealthy in vegetables. To some degree, this impact might be ascribed to cell reinforcements (nutrients C and E, selenium, and carotenoids).

4) Vegetables are a definitive food substitution. Adding supplement thick food sources like vegetables, which are plentiful in fiber, cell reinforcements, and nutrients, to your eating routine can cause you to feel improved and get in shape. Low quality food and handled starches are stacked with unfortunate fats and lacking in supplements.

5) Vegetables assist you with getting more fit. Vegetables are low in calories, however they keep up with your wellbeing and save you more full for a more

extended timeframe. Assuming you eat entire food varieties and keep away from bundled food varieties and food sources without supplements, you might eat less calories regardless feel fulfilled.

Natural products YOU Ought to Stay away from FOR Weight reduction

1. Bananas

Bananas aren't awful. A medium banana contains around 3 grams of fiber and tolerably affects glucose. However, there are a great deal of natural products that are better. Also, bananas can undoubtedly be abused while designating your day to day organic product recompense.
All things considered, avocados are an extraordinary other option. These can assist you with accomplishing similar richness as bananas in smoothies. They are loaded with solid fats that can assist with easing back the assimilation of sugars and keep you full.
2. Dried Natural products

Dried natural products sound like a solid tidbit. Sadly, they spike your glucose far more than normal organic product, which assists you with putting away fat. Furthermore, this can be a major issue in the event that you're hoping to shed a couple of pounds.
All things being equal, go for trail blend. Attempt crude cacao nibs rather than dried natural products in your blend. The crude cacao will contain some normal pleasantness. Also, it can assist individuals with glucose issues!
3. Papayas

Papaya's effect on glucose is on the better quality for natural products. What's more, they score lower on fiber count. In this way, you will need to keep papaya utilization in

Control. All things being equal, attempt a nectarine. Nectarines modest affect glucose. Furthermore, they are a decent wellspring of potassium and L-ascorbic acid.

4. Pineapples

A pineapple is unfortunately another delicious, cooling organic product that isn't as weight reduction well disposed. Pineapple is high in sugar, which is presumably why it is utilized as a treat or for the sake of entertainment drinks like Pina Coladas. All things being equal, attempt a crude coconut, which has an unpretentious pleasantness. With some restraint, it is an incredible wellspring of solid fats. Furthermore, very much like pineapple, it can make an extraordinary consummation of a feast.

5. Mangoes

Nothing can truly be said about mangoes that haven't previously been said to describe other delicious organic products. They are high in sugar and are best consumed with some restraint while attempting to get more fit. All things being equal, attempt a peach. Peaches affect glucose. What's more, they are great wellsprings of vitamin A, nutrient C, and potassium.

1. **Fruit Juice**

Fruit juice is everything problematic about juicy fruits brought to the extreme. Whenyou separate fruit sugar from fruit fiber, you get a glass of fruit-flavored sugar. Fruit juice, thus made, can be almost as problematic for weight loss as soda.

Instead, try a nice green vegetable juice instead. You'll save your waistline and get all the vitamins and minerals you need. Drinking green vegetable juice can boost your nutrient intake, which will not only boost your metabolism but also toneyour entire body.

VEGETABLES YOU SHOULD AVOID FOR WEIGHT LOSS

1. Pumpkins

Pumpkins should be consumed in moderation while trying to lose weight, as they can really spike your blood sugar. And when your blood sugar goes up, you're likelyto start packing on the pounds. Instead, eat sweet potatoes, which have a smaller impact on blood sugar. They're also high in many nutrients like carotenoids, B

Vitamins and vitamin A. Use them instead of pumpkin stews, casseroles, andother dishes.

2. White Potato

White potatoes will do more than just spike your blood sugar. They will leave you undernourished. White potatoes really lack the nutrients of their veggie brethren. So,instead, try baked zucchini chips instead of potato chips. Just add a little olive oil and salt, and bake. Zucchini is kinder on the waistline. Plus, it is a good source of vitaminC, vitamin B, and magnesium.

3. Corn

Not only is corn a starchier, more fattening vegetable, but also very likely to be genetically modified. The effect of such foods on the body and metabolism is still under much debate. But don't go crying over giving up your corn tortillas. Instead,try coconut flour tortillas. You can buy them from specialty stores or make them yourself if you have a press.

4. Parsnips

The glycemic load of a parsnip is worse than a white potato, which means it will spikeyour blood sugar and really make you pack on the pounds. This is kind of crazy for a healthy-sounding veggie. It's also not as nutritionally rich as many other veggies.

So, instead, try celery root instead of parsnips in your favorite recipes. Celery root is high in fiber as well as nutrients like potassium and magnesium. Not to mention, it isvery helpful in losing weight.

5. Beets

Beets are healthy foods but don't eat them too often while trying to lose weight. Theyare starchy vegetables and can make you gain weight. Instead, get all the nutrition from beets without the starch. Use beet greens in recipes. Phosphorus, zinc, and vitamin B-6 are all found in high concentrations in them, and they are low in starch.

6. Carrots

Carrots are naturally higher in starch and sugar. You can eat them in moderation, but if you're trying to lose weight, don't make them your main choice. Instead, go for celery when you want something crunchy. Celery has virtuallyno calories and is a source of nutrients like B vitamins, calcium, and magnesium.

Fruits and vegetables can be a supportive part of any weight loss diet. Just make sureyou're eating the right ones and focusing on the most helpful ones to reach your goals. Limit the ones that will just leave your weight-loss dreams in the dust.

To reap the full benefits offered by fruits and vegetables, keep in mind that you should have various types of these. Let your plate be colorful, and make sure you aregetting enough!

EAT HEALTHY TO FEEL HEALTHY

Have you heard the old saying which says, "you are what you eat?

Most people don't think about what they put into their bodies. In fact, there is a phrase for it called "mindless eating" by Brian Wansink in a book bearing the same name. According to Wansink, we make more than 200 food decisions every single day, and yet we are unaware of 90 percent of them. That means we make 180 passivefood-related decisions every single day.

If you are looking to lose weight, what you eat is extremely important. There are certain foods that help you lose weight more effectively than others, and if you want to be successful, you need tomake sure you are eating the right things. Eating a healthy diet will help you lose weight and keep it off.

Eating a variety of healthy foods is part of a weight management plan. You can think of eating the rainbow by adding a variety of colors to your plate. Vitamins, fiber, and minerals are abundant in dark, leafy greens, oranges, and tomatoes. Stews, omelets, and soups can be instantly boosted with color and nutrients by adding frozen peppers, broccoli, or onions.

The Dietary Guidelines for Americans 2020–2025 pdf icon [PDF-30.6MB]externalicon recommends the following healthy eating plan:

- Promotes the consumption of fruits, vegetables, whole grains, and dairy products with low fat or no fat
- There are many different protein foods to choose from, including seafood (seafood and fish), lean meat, poultry, eggs, beans, peas, soy, nuts, and seeds.
- There are no calories, trans fats, saturated fats, or cholesterol in it.
- Consume a healthy amount of calories each day

FRUIT

Canned, frozen, or fresh fruits are all good options. Mango, pineapple, and kiwi fruit are fruit alternatives to apples and bananas. For fruit that isn't in season, freeze it, can it, or dry it. Added sugars and syrups may be present in dried and canned fruit. Canning fruit in water or in its own juice is a good choice.

VEGETABLES

With an herb like rosemary, you can add a new flavor to grilled or steamed vegetables. A small amount of cooking spray can also be used to sauté (panfry) vegetables. Or make a quick side dish with frozen or canned vegetables. Don't forget to look for canned vegetables that aren't seasoned, flavored, or topped with butter or cream. Keep a variety of vegetables on hand by trying a new one each week.

CALCIUM-RICH FOODS

Consider low-fat and fat-free yogurts without added sugar in addition to fat-free and low-fat milk. You can substitute these for desserts because they come in a variety of flavors.

Increasing calcium intake alone may not help in weight loss, but when combinedwith dairy protein, it definitely translates to weight loss.

However, you can acquire calcium from non-dairy sources to it.

Calcium is an essential nutrient not only for weight loss but also to preserve bone health, dental health, and even for something as small as cellular reactions.

Ensure you are getting your healthy dose of calcium.

MEATS

You can make healthier versions of your favorite recipes by baking or grilling fish or chicken instead of frying them. Alternatively, you can use dry beans instead of meat. Try searching for calorie-free recipes online and in magazines. You may discover a new favorite!

COMFORT FOODS

photo of 2 variations of macaroni and cheese, one with 540 calories and one with 315calories

It's all about balance when it comes to healthy eating. No matter how high in calories, fat, or sugar your favorite foods are, you can still enjoy them. You can eat them occasionally if you follow a healthy diet and exercise regularly.

Generally, comfort foods should be prepared as follows:

- Reduce the frequency of eating them. Reduce your intake of these foods to once or twice a month if you normally eat them every day.
- Reduce the amount of food you eat. You can cut the size of or only eat half a chocolate bar if that is your favorite high-calorie food.
- Consider a version with fewer calories. Prepare your food differently or choose ingredients with fewer calories.
- You can reduce the fat in your mac and cheese by substituting nonfat milk, less butter, low-fat cheese, fresh spinach, and tomatoes. Just make sure not to increase your portion size.

I've prepared a list of easy-to-prepare and combination foods that are great for weight loss. Just add these overachievers to your grocery list now, and you'll be glad you did.

1. Whole Eggs

It's safe to assume that eggs made the cut already, right? It's true that eggs are a heavy-weight-loss classic, but as well as keeping your belly full, they will also keep your batteries charged!

The popularity of eggs in weight loss has grown after they were once viewed as a food that could raise bad LDL cholesterol. In addition to being inexpensive, easy to prepare, and available, they are excellent weight-loss foods.

Breakfast or brunch with high-protein foods, such as a veggie omelet or poached egg on toast, can provide much-needed energy during the day. You can even keep yourself full until dinner by eating hard-boiled eggs atop a delicious salad.

2. Leafy Greens

Making dietary changes that include more leafy greens, such as eating more leafy greens, can help you shed those extra pounds.

There are many superfoods loaded with fiber, vitamins, and minerals, such as spinach, kale, lettuce, cabbage, and microgreens. This side dish or salad ingredient is perfect for adding to salads.

Incorporating leafy greens into your diet will add volume to your meals while reducing calories. You'll feel full all day long and will not feel guilty about treating yourself to a big lunch.

3. Fatty Fish

A nice fillet of fatty fish is a great way to get some healthy protein. Salmon, tuna, and sardines are great choices due to their omega-3 content and lean protein content. Salmon is an excellent dinner choice because of its unsaturated fatty acids and minerals.

Vitamin D is also found in salmon and may help control weight, according to research. As well as containing 25% of your daily vitamin B6, salmon is also good for regulating your mood and stress levels.

It will help you avoid unwanted cravings later in the day or at night if you eat fatty fish during the day. When it comes to losing weight, I recommend this food.

4. Apple Cider Vinegar

Natural product juice is all that risky about delicious organic products brought to the limit. At the point when you separate organic product sugar from organic product fiber, you get a glass of organic product seasoned sugar. Natural product juice, accordingly made, can be nearly as tricky for weight reduction as pop.
All things considered, attempt a decent green vegetable juice all things considered. You'll save your waistline and get every one of the nutrients and minerals you really want. Drinking green vegetable juice can support your supplement consumption, which won't just lift your digestion yet in addition tone your whole body.

VEGETABLES YOU Ought to Keep away from FOR Weight reduction

1.   Pumpkins

Pumpkins ought to be consumed with some restraint while attempting to get more fit, as they
can truly spike your glucose. What's more, when your glucose goes up, you're probably going to begin pressing on the pounds. All things considered, eat yams, which smallerly affect glucose. They're additionally high in numerous supplements like carotenoids, B

Nutrients and vitamin A. Use them rather than pumpkin stews, goulashes, and different dishes.
2.   White Potato

White potatoes will accomplish something beyond spike your glucose. They will leave you undernourished. White potatoes truly miss the mark on supplements of their veggie brethren. In this way, all things being equal, attempt heated zucchini chips rather than potato chips. Simply add a little olive oil and salt, and heat. Zucchini is kinder on the waistline. Furthermore, it is a decent wellspring of L-ascorbic acid, vitamin B, and magnesium.
3.   Corn

In addition to the fact that corn is a starchier, really swelling vegetable, yet in addition prone to be hereditarily changed. The impact of such food varieties on the body and digestion is still under much discussion. In any case, don't go

crying over surrendering your corn tortillas. All things considered, attempt coconut flour tortillas. You can get them from specialty stores or make them yourself in the event that you have a press.
4.   Parsnips

The glycemic heap of a parsnip is more terrible than a white potato, and that implies it will spike your glucose and truly make you pack on the pounds. This is somewhat insane for a solid sounding veggie. It's additionally not so healthfully rich as numerous different veggies.
Along these lines, all things being equal, attempt celery root rather than parsnips in your number one recipes. Celery root is high in fiber as well as supplements can imagine potassium and magnesium. Also, it is extremely useful in shedding pounds.
5.   Beets

Beets are good food sources yet don't eat them time and again while attempting to get more fit. They are bland vegetables and can make you put on weight. All things being equal, get all the nourishment from beets without the starch. Use beet greens in recipes. Phosphorus, zinc, and vitamin B-6 are undeniably tracked down in high focuses in them, and they are low in starch.
6.   Carrots

Carrots are normally higher in starch and sugar. You can eat them with some restraint, yet assuming that you're attempting to get in shape, don't pursue them your principal decision. All things considered, go for celery when you need something crunchy. Celery has for all intents and purposes no calories and is a wellspring of supplements like B nutrients, calcium, and magnesium.

Foods grown from the ground can be a steady piece of any weight reduction diet. Simply ensure you're eating the right ones and zeroing in on the most supportive ones to arrive at your objectives. Limit the ones that will simply leave your weight reduction dreams in the residue.

To receive the full rewards presented by foods grown from the ground, remember that you ought to have different kinds of these. Allow your plate to be vivid, and ensure you are getting enough!

EAT Beneficial TO FEEL Great

Have you heard the familiar axiom which says, "for getting healthy, the kind of food you eat is everything?

A great many people don't ponder what they put into their bodies. Truth be told, there is an expression for it called "careless eating" by Brian Wansink in a book bearing a similar name. As per Wansink, we go with in excess of 200 food choices each and every day, but we know nothing about 90% of them. That implies we go with 180 latent food-related choices each and every day.

In the event that you are hoping to get in shape, what you eat is critical. There are sure food sources that assist you with shedding pounds more actually than others, and to find success, you really want to ensure you are eating the right things. Eating a sound eating routine will assist you with shedding pounds and keep it off.

Eating various good food sources is essential for a weight the board plan. You can imagine eating the rainbow by changing it up of varieties to your plate. Nutrients, fiber, and minerals are plentiful in dull, mixed greens, oranges, and tomatoes. Stews, omelets, and soups can be right away helped with variety and supplements by adding frozen peppers, broccoli, or onions.

The Dietary Rules for Americans 2020-2025 pdf symbol [PDF-30.6MB]externalicon suggests the accompanying smart dieting plan:
•   Advances the utilization of organic products, vegetables, entire grains, and dairy items with low fat or no fat
•   There are a wide range of protein food sources to browse, including fish (fish and fish), lean meat, poultry, eggs, beans, peas, soy, nuts, and seeds.
•   There are no calories, trans fats, soaked fats, or cholesterol in it.
•   Consume a sound measure of calories every day

Natural product

Canned, frozen, or new natural products are great choices. Mango, pineapple, and kiwi natural product are organic product options in contrast to apples and bananas. For natural product that isn't in season, freeze it, can it, or dry it. Added sugars and syrups might be available in dried and canned organic product. Canning natural product in water or in its own juice is a decent decision.

VEGETABLES

With a spice like rosemary, you can add another flavor to barbecued or steamed vegetables. A modest quantity of cooking shower can likewise be utilized to sauté (sear) vegetables. Or on the other hand make a fast side dish with frozen or canned vegetables. Remember to search for canned vegetables that aren't prepared, seasoned, or finished off with margarine or cream. Keep various vegetables close by attempting another one every week.

CALCIUM-RICH Food sources

Consider low-endlessly fat free yogurts without added sugar notwithstanding sans fat and low-fat milk. You can substitute these for treats since they arrive in different flavors.
Expanding calcium admission alone may not help in weight reduction, but rather when joined with dairy protein, it certainly means weight reduction. Notwithstanding, you can obtain calcium from non-dairy sources to it.

Calcium is a fundamental supplement for weight reduction as well as to save bone wellbeing, dental wellbeing, and in any event, for something as little as cell responses.
Guarantee you are getting your solid portion of calcium.

MEATS

You can make better renditions of your number one recipes by baking or barbecuing fish or chicken as opposed to broiling them. Then again, you can utilize dry beans rather than meat. Have a go at looking for without calorie recipes on the web and in magazines. You might find another number one!

Solace Food varieties

photograph of 2 varieties of macaroni and cheddar, one with 540 calories and one with 315 calories
Everything unquestionably revolves around balance with regards to good dieting. Regardless of how high in calories, fat, or sugar your number one food sources are, you can in any case appreciate them. You can eat them infrequently on the off chance that you follow a solid eating regimen and work-out consistently.

By and large, solace food sources ought to be ready as follows:
*   Decrease the recurrence of eating them. Decrease your admission of these

food varieties to on more than one occasion per month assuming that you ordinarily eat them consistently.

•	Diminish how much food you eat. You can cut the size of or possibly eat a portion of a chocolate bar assuming that that is your #1 fatty food.

•	Think about a variant with less calories. Set up your food contrastingly or pick fixings with less calories.

•	You can diminish the fat in your macintosh and cheddar by subbing nonfat milk, less spread, low-fat cheddar, new spinach, and tomatoes. Simply make a point not to build your part size.

I've arranged a rundown of simple to-get ready and mix food sources that are perfect for weight reduction. Simply add these overachievers to your staple rundown now, and you'll be happy you did.

1.	Whole Eggs

It's most likely the case that eggs got it done as of now, correct? The facts really confirm that eggs are a significant burden misfortune exemplary, however as well as keeping your tummy full, they will likewise keep your batteries charged!

The prominence of eggs in weight reduction has developed after they were once seen as a food that could raise terrible LDL cholesterol. As well as being cheap, simple to get ready, and accessible, they are amazing weight reduction food sources.

Breakfast or early lunch with high-protein food varieties, like a veggie omelet or poached egg on toast, can give genuinely necessary energy during the day. You might in fact keep yourself full until supper by eating hard-bubbled eggs on a scrumptious serving of mixed greens.

2.	Leafy Greens

Rolling out dietary improvements that incorporate more mixed greens, like eating more salad greens, can assist you with shedding those additional pounds. There are numerous superfoods stacked with fiber, nutrients, and minerals, like spinach, kale, lettuce, cabbage, and microgreens. This side dish or salad fixing is ideal for adding to plates of mixed greens.
Integrating salad greens into your eating routine will add volume to your dinners while diminishing calories. You'll feel full the entire day and won't feel remorseful about indulging yourself with a major lunch.

3.   Fatty Fish

A pleasant filet of greasy fish is an incredible method for getting some solid protein. Salmon, fish, and sardines are incredible decisions because of their omega-3 substance and lean protein content. Salmon is an amazing supper decision in view of its unsaturated fats and minerals.
Vitamin D is additionally viewed as in salmon and may assist with controlling weight, as per research. As well as containing 25% of your everyday vitamin B6, salmon is additionally really great for directing your mind-set and feelings of anxiety.
It will assist you with staying away from undesirable desires later in the day or around evening time in the event that you eat greasy fish during the day. With regards to getting in shape, I suggest this food.

5. Apple Juice Vinegar

It's valid: Apple juice vinegar is respected by the sound way of life local area.

There are many advantages to utilizing this wellbeing tonic. In examinations, it has been

displayed to further develop digestion, control hunger, and keep up with glucose levels.

One to two tablespoons of this 'remedy' each day are suggested. It very well may be eaten

before a feast or blended in with a few water and prepared on a plate of mixed greens.

Consistently passes, and the yearning dies down.

6.   Nuts

Since nuts come in such wide assortments, you might find it hard to tell which nuts are best for

your eating regimen. They are a decent wellspring of monosaturated fats that make them

heart-sound tidbits. You could supplant chips and pretzels with nuts assuming you used to go

after those all things considered.

In any case, on the off chance that you should try not to nibble in that frame of mind no matter

what, simply toss a couple into your morning shake. A few human examinations have shown

that individuals who consistently consume nuts are fitter and more grounded than the people

who don't, generally because of the nuts' impact on supercharging digestion systems.

7.   Quinoa

The wellbeing food office is notable for its quinoa items. There's no gluten in it, and it's stacked with fiber and protein. The nine fundamental amino acids it contains make it an uncommon wellspring of protein.
You will remain full for longer and eat less unfortunate bites assuming that you consume these properties of the quinoa seeds. Besides, it has a low glycemic record, which is perfect for glucose levels since it doesn't thoroughly upset them.

8.   Avocado

As the gold medalist of the solid fats Olympics, avocados are in vogue, famous, and loaded with medical advantages. Avocados are viewed as weight reduction champions for various reasons. The fats, fiber, and water in avocados make them a sound option in contrast to most natural products that are high in starches. In view of these qualities, they are low in energy thickness and are a magnificent fat-consuming food.
Feeling somewhat exhausted with your serving of mixed greens? Avocados add a ton of flavor to any dish. You've recently found another superfood that can assist you with getting more fit assuming you keep it moderate.

9.   Citrus Natural products

Is it challenging for you to practice since you feel depleted? How might your temperament be worked on by a little daylight? You've come to the perfect locations in the event that you are searching for food to reestablish your energy.
Notwithstanding their nutrient substance, citrus organic products like lemons, oranges, limes, grapefruits, and others contain fiber, water, and fiber. Moreover, they are high in potassium, which lessens swelling, and they contain cancer prevention agents, which battle irritation.

10.   Peanut Spread

Did you realize peanut butter made this rundown?

Fortunately peanut butter keeps you feeling full and fulfilled over the course of the day, whether you like it smooth or thick.

A serving of this food has as much as 8 grams of protein and 4 grams of fiber, going with it a phenomenal decision for counts calories that plan to shed pounds.

The explanation peanut butter can assist you with getting thinner is that it holds your glucose levels consistent, kills yearning, and controls your hunger.

11.   Full-Fat Greek Yogurt

A lot of interest is right now being given to Greek yogurt, and that is absolutely reasonable! Have you at any point asked why?

There is proof to help the possibility that full-fat yogurt can assist you with shedding pounds more really than low-fat dairy products.[5] The probiotic properties of unsweetened full-fat yogurt can be valuable for supporting invulnerability, directing stomach capability, and lessening bulging and liquid maintenance.

Leptin (the chemical that manages craving, weight, and digestion) is more averse to be impervious to leptin in people with solid guts. Ensure the yogurt you pick is full-fat and contains something like five dynamic societies. Most of different yogurts are stacked with sugar and contain basically no probiotics.

12.   Berries

As far as fiber content, berries are very high. Among the most well known natural products are blueberries and raspberries. There are around 6-8 grams of fiber in a cup of berries, and fiber is referred to assist with overseeing weight as well as energy levels.

As a tidbit or treat, they go with an extraordinary decision since they're solid, low in sugar, and taste perfect. To make an even breakfast that is sound and reviving, include strong cell reinforcement properties.

You will feel like you are getting a treat for body and soul in the event that you consolidate a few boundaries with Greek yogurt toward the beginning of the day.

13.   Herbs and Flavors

Work on your figure however tired of plain, exhausting food? Does each sound decision taste terrible? My story is totally different from yours!
You don't need to sentence your taste buds to death to deal with your wellbeing. You will lose all disdain for eating less junk food the second you add some really preparing. The spice and flavor rack is ideal over the salt shaker (sodium is water-holding and causes bulging).

I like to utilize the accompanying flavors:
•   basil
•   cilantro
•   cinnamon
•   rosemary
•   curry
•   cumin
•   oregano
•   ginger
•   dark pepper

14.   Dark chocolate

The best is on the way! The utilization of dim chocolate might add to weight reduction, as per a few examinations. This can assist you with getting thinner by diminishing desires and advancing sensations of completion. [6]

The superfood's capacity to further develop insulin responsiveness, lift mind-set, and lift energy affirms its status as a rising star. However long you don't overdo it on dim chocolate, dim chocolate is the ideal nibble for those with a sweet tooth.

It is not difficult to pick the best food varieties to eat for weight reduction since there are such countless choices. You won't need to stress over taking your sound fats and proteins, strands, cell reinforcements, nutrients, and minerals on the off chance that your shopping basket is loaded down with lean protein, new leafy foods, nuts, and entire grains. These supplements produce energy inside the cells, support your safe framework, and assist you with getting more fit.

Plunk DOWN AND EAT

We're generally in a hurry. The measurements for the number of feasts Americans that eat in the vehicle are continually expanding, and it's very upsetting. We're in such a rush that we'll eat food that is horrible as far as we're concerned basically for happiness, however we eat it so quick that we scarcely appreciate it. One explanation we indulge is a direct result of the time defer between our body handling what we've eaten and conveying that completion message to our cerebrum.

Your body is intended to eat at a specific speed, so when you eat quicker than that, when your body feels full, you've previously eaten for 10 additional minutes than you ought to have. Your stomach is 50% or 60% overstuffed on the grounds that you didn't give your body sufficient opportunity to convey that message.

One of the principles of careful eating is to arrive at a condition of complete focus with the food you put into your body. It requires around 20 minutes for your cerebrum to understand that you're full. To this end you need to loosen up the feasting experience. As indicated by Zane Andrews, an academic administrator of physiology and a neuroscientist at Monash College, when we put food into our mouths, we promptly get the sign that it's delectable, and this makes a longing to eat more.

In any case, it's not until food arrives at the stomach that it begins to deliver the chemicals that let us know we're full. It requires 5 to 20 minutes for the food to be handled sufficient that our stomach delivers those chemicals. Our bodies were intended to lean toward indulging since we come from a universe of endurance. A portion of quite a while back, eating quicker and indulging would give you the additional energy you expected to battle a tiger. Our bodies haven't advanced for our new climate where the risk comes from indulging instead of under-eating.

Like careful eating, careful eating concentrates to what you consume. Focus on the smell, the flavors, and the surface of the food as opposed to eating missing mindedly. Try not to browse your email or virtual entertainment on your telephone as opposed to being completely present in the

Process of eating. Every bite and every sip should be deliberate. In simplest terms,mindful eating is consuming food with intention.

According to healthline.com, there are a host of benefits to mindful eating:

1. Over 85 percent of obese individuals who lose weight return to (or exceed) theirinitial weight loss within a few years.
2. Mindful eating helps you to lose weight by changing your eating behaviors and reducing stress. Because mindful eating changes the way you think about food, and it's a way of life rather than a diet, it's maintainable. When you lose weight, followingthis method helps the weight stay off.
3. Unlike a diet you activate when you want to lose weight and turn off when you hit your goals, mindful eating is a continuous and permanent process. Just changing theway you think about food allows you to remove many of the negative feelings that you associate with eating and replace them with awareness, improved self-control, and positive emotions. Mindful eating has been shown to dramatically reduce the severity and frequency of binge eating.
4. Mindful eating reduces emotional eating. Rather than responding to internal cues based on how you're feeling in that moment (such as when someone hurts your feelings or you have a bad day) or external cues (such as sight, smell, commercials,and peer pressure), you'll now eat based on conscious decisions.

So, does mindful eating sound like a habit that will help with your weight loss journey? If so, then there are a few strategies you can use to build this practice.

HOW TO EAT MINDFULLY

There are several strategies you can put into place to make mindful eating an easyand consistent part of your life:

1. Build junk food barriers.

As per Wansink, we eat what we find in our current circumstance. That incorporates treats, frozen yogurt, and bites. A hankering for guilty pleasure is almost difficult to oppose, so the most secure thing you can do isn't buy that stuff when you are at the supermarket.

Along these lines, on the off chance that you long for unfortunate, calorie-filled snacks, you need to get in the vehicle and go to the store as opposed to just strolling across the kitchen.
This standard applies to your working environment also. Try not to stock an individual region with low quality food. The last thing you really want is a cabinet loaded up with treats and undesirable tidbits enticing you over the course of the day.
You really want to include procedures to forestall enticement and openness to inactive exercises or social eating. We eat despite the fact that we aren't ravenous; we hit up gatherings and occasions where everybody is eating; we head out to films where it appears to be simply normal to stir things up around town stand notwithstanding the over the top costs.
Limit the amount you go to occasions like these to diminish how frequently you need to confront these allurements. Your cabinet ought to be loaded with food sources and tidbits that are solid, and they ought to be food varieties that you appreciate eating. Like that, you don't have the compulsion to bounce in your vehicle and drive to a cheap food joint when your belly begins thundering.
2.   Eat gradually.

One of the fundamentals of careful eating is to arrive at a condition of undivided focus with the food you put into your body. It requires around 20 minutes for your cerebrum to understand that you're full. For this reason you need to loosen up the feasting experience.
As indicated by Zane Andrews, an academic partner of physiology and a neuroscientist at Monash College, when we put food into our mouths, we quickly get the sign that it's scrumptious, and this makes a craving to eat more. Nonetheless, it's not until food arrives at the stomach that it begins to deliver the chemicals that let us know we're full. It requires 5 to 20 minutes for the food to be handled sufficient that our stomach delivers those chemicals. Our bodies were intended to incline toward indulging since we come from a universe of endurance. A portion of quite a while back, eating quicker and indulging would give you the additional energy you expected to battle a tiger. Our bodies haven't developed for our new climate where the peril comes from indulging instead of

under-eating.
- Eating gradually gives your body time to let you know when it's full, and there are different ways of carrying out this cycle:

- Eat-in a climate that is without interruption. Try not to sit in front of the TV, read, or take a gander at your telephone while you're eating. This is something contrary to careful eating.
- Take a stab at eating with others. This can dial back the eating system as you're taken part in discussion.
- Put down your cutlery between each nibble.
- Eat high-fiber food varieties and require a long time to bite.
- Taste water between each nibble.
- Count the quantity of messes with you take of each piece of food. Building up to 20 preceding you swallow will dial back your eating pace and power you to remain in a condition of care.

3.   Pay regard for your faculties in general.

Racing through a feast — particularly a dinner that is terrible for you — is such a waste. We're in such a hurry to put something horrendous for us into our bodies, and we don't for a moment even find opportunity to partake in the wrongdoing. Carve out opportunity to appreciate all that you eat with however many faculties as would be prudent. Notice the varieties, shut your eyes, partake in the fragrance of the food, and value the kinds of each chomp. How can it feel in your mouth? What do you appreciate about it?
Whether eating something solid or unfortunate, partaking in the process will keep you in a condition of care. On the off chance that you require some investment to partake in your dinner, you're fighting the temptation to heap food into your mouth, and you hold eating back from turning into a mechanical cycle.

4.   Understand your singular food cravings.

A careless dietary pattern is not difficult to create. That is the reason you really want to comprehend your body-explicit signs for when you're eager and when you're essentially exhausted and searching for something to do.
- Do you feel an unfilled gut?
- Do you feel your stomach snarling?
- Do you encounter tipsiness, thirst, or low energy?

Assuming you know when you're eager, you can isolate that from when you want to eat in light of the fact that you have nothing else to do. You'll be better prepared to answer flags that your body's sending you.

5.   Sit down at a table.

Eating at the feasting table makes a condition of care, and it's the best spot you can eat. Sitting in your vehicle or sitting on the love seat in your front room — those are where we are probably going to eat without care and without center. We can over-eat, indulge, and eat undesirable tidbits when we aren't focusing on the thing we're doing.

We need to eat to turn into a functioning movement. Very much like your bed ought to just be for resting, you need to make a spot that is just for eating so your psyche realizes that this is where you center around eating. Your body will hope to be in an interruption free perspective.

Work on EATING Carefully WITH OTHERS

Assuming that you're encircled by others, and you attempt to rehearse your standard careful eating rehearses where you're centered altogether around the thing you're eating, you'll disregard individuals around you, and this can cause socially off-kilter circumstances.
You need to remain careful while taking part in the discussion with people around you. We have a few hints to help you through this interaction:
•   Ground yourself. As you're sitting in the seat, notice how it feels against your back and legs. When you stand on the ground, how can it feel? How do the utensils feel in your grasp? This will start to actuate those careful idea designs.
•   Request first. At the point when the server puts in the request, the remainder of the table follows, and on the off chance that you're not requesting first, you can be influenced into following the group as opposed to requesting what your body needs.

•   Go with what you know. Request something recognizable so you can zero in more energy on individuals around you as opposed to the subtleties of the new surfaces, flavors, and scents. Ask yourself, what's something that you can believe you'll appreciate, despite the fact that you can't be careful in that frame of mind to appreciate it?
•   Set the rhythm. It's not difficult to be impacted by how quick or slow individuals around the table are eating. Similarly as you will walk quicker to

stay aware of one of your companions, you will eat quicker to do precisely the same thing. Be that as it may, assuming you are deliberately eating more slow, you can be the person who establishes the vibe for the gathering.
•	Put down your fork and separate your chomps with discussion. While you're talking, put down the cutlery so you don't coincidentally eat in that frame of mind of the discussion. This will guarantee that you don't coincidentally eat without care.
•	Embrace doggie sacks. Anticipate extras. Surprisingly better, do what we recommended previously and request a portion of your dinner to place into a to-go holder. Along these lines, you're not enticed to eat assuming that you move pulled away from your care practice.
•	Pick your organization admirably. Whenever the situation allows, the discussion can upgrade the careful eating practice insight. Be that as it may, on the off chance that it's critical, you need to move the discussion completely away from food.

In the event that you want to, get some information about loved ones as opposed to discussing diets and bodies. The last thing you need is for everybody around the table to take a gander at you and spotlight on the thing you're doing. This will divert you from careful eating and make you bound to submit to enticement when the remainder of the table chooses to arrange a treat.

A SIMPLE MINDFUL EATING EXERCISE

To integrate this segment, we should discuss a straightforward careful eating exercise that depends on crafted by John Kabat-Zinn.
The advantages of this exercise are that it diminishes impulsive eating exercises brought about by feeling, improves your familiarity with food decisions, increments the amount you appreciate eating, and assists you with fortifying the muscle of presence as opposed to that of distraction.

To begin, track down a little nibble as raisins, natural product, popcorn, or peanuts.

Then, get into a familiar situated position and come into the current second by taking a couple of breaths. Focus on how all aspects of your body feels.
Place a couple of raisins in your grasp and notice the impulse to place that small bunch into your mouth. Oppose that enticement, take a gander at every

individual raisin, and look at them with a condition of interest like you've never seen a raisin. Attempt to see how every raisin is not quite the same as the others — very much like snowflakes; each raisin is remarkable.

Focus on how they feel in your grasp — the surface, the shape, the weight, and the appearance. You might need to shut your eyes while doing this, so you can zero in on different components and get further into what makes this raisin novel.

Move past the current second and envision where the raisins came from and how they began as grapes on the plant. Envision the specialists culling those grapes, moving them into a container, conveying them into the horse shelter, and, over the long haul, the rancher concluding that these grapes would be better off as raisins. Envision the method involved with drying them out and changing over them into the raisins you see before you now.

After this psychological activity, gradually carry a solitary raisin to your nose, smell it, and recognize the bouquet. Notice how normally your arm moves to play out this activity, and keep on seeing any considerations you have, whether they're positive or negative, about this raisin.

Might it be said that you are guessing what it will suggest a flavor like? Could it be said that you are beginning to salivate?

Could it be said that you are feeling a motivation to place the raisin into your mouth immediately?

Remain in a condition of care, in unlimited oversight, and spot the primary raisin in your mouth. Without gnawing it, investigate what it seems like in your mouth. Notice what your tongue is doing. Save it in your mouth without biting for no less than 10 seconds. You need to encounter the taste and surface without biting for an entire 10 seconds.

At the point when you're prepared, gradually and delicately start to nibble into the raisin, taking a solitary chomp. Presently, without gulping, notice what it has an aftertaste like as it's torn open, how the flavor

What's more, surface changes as you bite. Notice and oppose your normal drive to swallow it. Just when you are prepared, and it is a cognizant choice, do you swallow.

Sit discreetly and remain at the time as you notice what you're feeling, and afterward rehash with the following raisin. This is an action you could attempt with other little, scaled down food varieties like popcorn, peanuts, or other little natural products. All things considered, we've currently covered each of the four points of support you can use to dominate your dietary patterns. You presently know how to control what you put into your body through careful eating, key preparation, and the supplanting of undesirable food sources with solid ones. So how about we continue on toward the fifth and last propensity for this cycle — how to consolidate practice with savvy food choices.

Center Around THE Objective FOR YOUR Wellbeing

For what reason would it be a good idea for you to hold on until you are confronted with a perilous wellbeing emergency to need wellbeing greatness? The vast majority would decide to infection resistant their bodies and look extraordinary at this point. They simply never figured they could make it happen with such ease. Envision yourself in extraordinary wellbeing and in amazing state of being at your ideal body weight. Not exclusively will your abdomen be liberated from fat, however your heart will be liberated from plaque.

In any case, it isn't not difficult to change: eating has profound and social hints. Breaking an addiction is particularly troublesome. As you will learn, our American eating regimen style is habit-forming however not quite so habit-forming as smoking cigarettes. Halting smoking is extremely hard, yet many actually succeed. I have heard many reasons throughout the long term, from smokers meaning to stop and at times even from bombed calorie counters. It isn't not difficult to Roll out any improvement. Clearly, the vast majority know whether they change their eating regimen enough and exercise, they can get more fit — yet they actually can't make it happen.

Indeed, even with individuals not set in stone to stop smoking, that's what I demand assuming they are confronted with huge business related pressure, have a contention, get in an auto crash, or experience some other disaster, they shouldn't return to smoking and utilize smoking as a pressure reliever. "It isn't the case different with your weight reduction — acknowledge no justifiable reason to tumble off the cart on your weight reduction venture. You can cause an adjustment of your weight provided that you allow your body a fair opportunity. Try not to say you will check it out. Try not to attempt; all things considered, genuinely promise to get everything done as well as possible.

At the point when you get hitched, does the strict figure or equity of the harmony inquire, "Do you pledge to check this individual out?" When individuals let me know they will check it out, I say they forget about it and you have previously chosen to fizzle. It takes in excess of an attempt to get thinner; it takes a responsibility. A responsibility is a commitment that you stay with, regardless.

Without that responsibility, you are ill-fated to come up short. Allow yourself an opportunity to succeed this time, as a matter of fact. Assuming you focus on the interaction, you won't just get more fit and will work on your wellbeing and change your life until the end of time.
Settle on a reasonable decision among progress and disappointment. It makes just three basic strides. One, purchase the book; two, read the book; three, commit the responsibility. The third step is the tough decision, however that is all it is — another decision.

A solid eating regimen is significant, not only with the end goal of weight reduction. It is also significant for keeping up with generally speaking wellbeing. It gives fundamental supplements, liquid, and energy for the body. It additionally gives sufficient micronutrients. Remembering these food varieties for your eating regimen is basic for your general wellbeing. Following a sound diet is fundamental. The most ideal way to build your body's wellbeing is to consume new foods grown from the ground and to eat an eating regimen wealthy in fiber. In any case, you ought to recall that you shouldn't overlook the significance of macronutrients and nutrients.

Practicing good eating habits isn't hard. The key is to eat the perfect proportion of calories and eats food sources that are wealthy in supplements. The vast majority will quite often gorge, and they will more often than not indulge specific food sources. For instance, on the off chance that you eat an enormous part of pizza, you ought to eat more organic product. On the other hand, on the off chance that you're keen on keeping a thin and sound constitution, you ought to eat food sources that are low in calories.

There are numerous delectable and quality food sources that are low in fat. The most ideal way to keep your body solid is to eat a ton of foods grown from the ground. These are nutritious as well as extremely delectable. You can set up your own feasts and try not to eat handled food. Simple suppers you can make in minutes; have a go at planning feasts with organic products, vegetables, and nuts. Beside that, you ought as far as possible yourself from sweet and pungent food.

Quality food sources ought to be remembered for a reasonable eating regimen. A solid eating regimen is definitely not a set eating regimen. It's about equilibrium and balance. Counting a couple of treats is fine, however you ought to

Try not to eat a lot immediately. In the event that you're uncertain about whether a specific food is great for you, eating it in moderation is in every case better. It's critical to eat a solid eating routine that has a decent proportion of fat and protein to calories.

You ought to remember non-handled food varieties for your eating regimen notwithstanding good food sources. These sorts of food varieties are many times high in carbs, sugar, and fat. While you can't stay away from them altogether, you ought to restrict your admission of them. These food sources ought to be obtained from normal sources. They ought not be misleadingly enhanced. These food sources contain added substances that can possibly harm your body. Eat an assortment of without sugar and sans fat food sources to keep up with great wellbeing.

LET'S START WITH Disposing of SUGARS FROM YOUR Eating routine.

Science has found that a determined, raised insulin level is one of the primary drivers of corpulence, hypertension, and diabetes in this country. The utilization of fructose and sucrose in your eating regimen will incline you toward metabolic disorder (condition x), corpulence, diabetes, coronary illness (hypertension), and renal sickness. These sugars accelerate the illness by keeping up with different insulin spikes long after your dinner ought to have finished. Our bodies need glucose, which comes from vegetables and crude grains. Tenacious insulin spikes come from overabundance natural product sugars and synthetic or synthetically determined sugars like HFCS (high fructose corn syrup), sucrose, and fake sugars. Assuming we take a gander at the glycemic file (outlines and unites), we notice that fructose, sucrose, and other fructose compounds have critical readings, which ordinarily would show an insulin spike, however these sugars don't tie with insulin.

These types of sugar (fructose compounds and fake sugars) are just utilized by the liver, and extra insulin spikes happen after the glycogen is delivered by the liver (around one hour after the fact). These insulin spikes can be named auxiliary spikes, and they are the most harming to your wellbeing since they block your ghrelin reaction from your mind that would ordinarily stop hunger. Subsequently, your body

Convictions you are starving — and you continue to eat. The counterfeit sugars utilized today are fabricated materials or compound food sources that make hopeless harm the body straightforwardly.

If you look at the labels on the products in your pantry, the ingredients of 90 percent of these products contain toxic sugars. If your goal is to improve health, then eliminating these toxins must be your first move. Other foods that cause persistent insulin spikes are refined grains, gluten, whey, and the heavy starches found in potatoes and white rice (nonbondable fuels). Let's take a look at each to see why the foods that used to be so good for us are not so good now.

A diet rich in nutrients is important for maintaining a healthy weight. A diet rich in fiber, proteins, and fruits should be included in your daily meal. For instance, the consumption of sweets and chocolate should be restricted. You should limit the intake of unhealthy foods if you have diabetes. Instead, consume more fruit and vegetables, instead. If you're a vegetarian, eat plenty of nuts and whole-grain foods. Ifyou have diabetes, limit the intake of carbohydrates and fat.

It is so common these days for people to be on a tight schedule that they meet deadlines they rush around, forgetting about their health.

Our lives have become so fast-paced since we entered the digital age, get it quick mentalitythat we oftentimes skip and ignore some of the most important aspects of our life.

Healthful eating is often overlooked because it takes time and effort. In addition to heart disease, type 2 diabetes, high blood pressure, and obesity, neglecting this area of our lives contributes to their high incidence.

Let me first clarify that I'm not writing to criticize or guilt you into doing anything. Myself included, I have been guilty of neglecting my health more often than I should have.

It is my goal to change the way you think about eating healthy so that you realize how many positive effects eating healthy can have on your life. Healthier eating does more than just help you lose weight; here are a few things it does.

IMPROVES YOUR ENERGY LEVEL

Your energy level will skyrocket if you eat healthier foods. You get this effect from eating foods richer in vitamins B and D. You get more energy when you consume foods rich in these vitamins.

Furthermore, your body receives better types of carbohydrates and fats. To stay motivated, you need good fats (monounsaturated fats) and good carbohydrates (complex carbohydrates and resistant starches) while feeling unmotivated and tired from bad fats and sugars.

A future blog will explore the differences between fats and carbs in more detail.

REDUCES THE RISK OF DISEASES

The diet you choose can increase or reduce your risk of disease. Many people are unaware of how their eating habits can affect their health. Despite the fact that the following list is not exhaustive, it does provide a glimpse of some of the health issues that can arise as a result of ignoring your health. Dietary changes can reduce the risk of these conditions or improve their symptoms.

Macular degeneration and cataracts are two examples of eye diseases. Increasing free radical damage to the eyes is caused by a diet high in unhealthy foods. Fats that are commonly called bad fats, or trans-fats, are foods high in them and cause heart disease in some forms, whereas healthy foods are great for fighting off free radicals because they are antioxidant-rich. Taking omega-3 fatty acids and monounsaturated fats can improve the health of your heart.

A moderate consumption of dairy, fish, fruits, and vegetables can help prevent osteoporosis. The National Osteoporosis Foundation has recommended eating these foods in moderate amounts. The three main risk factors for type 2 diabetes are poor diet, obesity, and type 2 diabetes. By eating healthy, you will be able to eliminate these three risk factors as well as regulate your blood sugar levels, improve your energy, and enhance your brain function.

Boost Your Brain Function

Your brain will function better, and you will experience fewer mid-day crashes if your insulin and blood sugar levels are optimized. Eating fats and carbohydrates that are bad for you can affect the mood-regulating chemicals in your brain.

Several nutrients, including creatine, amino acids from grass-fed beef, omega-3 fatty acids from fish, and vitamin D from dairy, have been shown to boost moods and combat depression.

It Reduces Stress

Foods high in serotonin and dopamine help relax your body, and reduced cortisol levels reduce stress-inducing hormones. Your energy levels will stabilize when you eat balanced meals, and your energy levels won't dip as often during the day. You are more likely to stay on task if you have enough energy consistently, so you won't worry about forgetting something and making yourself stressed

Incorrectly doing something. Adding lean proteins to your diet can help you stay full and energy up throughout your day as egg whites, low-fat yogurt, fish, or soy. Having a consistent eating schedule and eating enough meals (i.e., not skipping meals) can once again help stabilize your energy levels. In addition to preventing you from overeating late in the day, eating small meals throughout the day will also prevent you from binge eating late in the day, which could lead to more stress because you feel guilty about overeating.

It Boosts Your Immunity

It is currently believed that eating healthy foods maintains healthy gut flora. By strengthening your immune system, you reduce your chances of contracting an infection. Nutrition can compromise the immune system by not providing enough energy and nutrients. Sarah Stanner, Science Director at the British Nutrition Foundation, says that no single nutrient, food, or supplement improves immunity or prevents infections like Covid-19.

When you choose foods that supply a steady stream of key nutrients, your immune system is best prepared to fight viruses. Whole plant foods, in particular, appear to stimulate the activity of natural killer cells. Natural killer cells are part of the innate immune system that targets pathogens, including viruses responsible for respiratory infections.

Immune System Booster Foods

Plant-based foods can strengthen the immune system because of their properties:
A mushroom's antioxidants and polysaccharides can enhance immunity and reduce inflammation, particularly in medicinal varieties like Chaga.
Brighter, the better when it comes to fruits and vegetables! Carotenoids, polyphenols, flavonoids, and anthocyanidins are phytochemicals with antioxidant and anti-inflammatory properties.
In support of proper T cell function and robust natural killer cell production, bitter greens like dandelion and arugula promote liver health.
A healthy gut requires fiber from whole grains and legumes. It's important to maintain a balanced gut because it's the major center of immune activity. B vitamins and zinc are also present in these foods, which help to boost the immune system.
Flax seeds are rich in omega-3 fatty acids, which are anti-inflammatory. Fat-soluble vitamins A, D, and E, which are essential for immune function, are also absorbed better through meals that include healthy fats.
Selenium, magnesium, and vitamin C are also essential nutrients for strengthening immunity. The best way to resist viruses and other pathogens is to build a strong immune system; it's important to eat a variety of whole-plant foods.

Foods That Weaken the Immune System

Viral infections are more likely to occur if you consume certain foods that weaken the immune system:

Inflammation is promoted by fried foods, dampening immunity in general.

The consumption of highly processed foods depletes nutrients and undermines the immune system.

You can have an immune system malfunction if you eat meat since it can contain food-borne pathogens, including viruses. Inflammation has also been shown to increase with many animal products.

All body systems can suffer serious consequences from these foods because they adversely affect gut health. Low fiber content combined with proinflammatory compounds skews the gut bacteria balance, resulting in weakened gut walls and chronic inflammation. Conversely, plant foods are generally anti-inflammatory and promote beneficial gut bacteria.

One powerful way to give your body the tools it needs to fight viruses is to switch your eating patterns away from processed and animal foods. You should also get enough sleep, exercise regularly, maintain a healthy stress level, and practice good hygiene so your immune system functions optimally. It is important to cultivate a healthy lifestyle to strengthen your immune system.

HELPS YOU LOSE WEIGHT

As discussed in the previous chapter, healthy eating is a key prerequisite for losing weight. Changing your diet from unhealthy to healthy will automatically result in weight loss. Weight loss doesn't require starving yourself. Don't worry.

Adding healthier foods to your diet will help you lose weight by supplying low-calorie, nutrient-dense calories. You don't need to restrict your calories at first. By substituting good calories for bad, you can reduce your calorie intake.

As your weight loss progresses, you can reduce your portion sizes.

IT LENGTHENS YOUR LIFE

You can naturally live a longer life if you eat healthily and avoid disease. An interesting fact to know is that eating seven or more servings of fruits and vegetables daily reduces the chance of keeling over by 42 percent compared to eating little or no produce.

It will take some time to adjust to the new lifestyle, so ignore the cravings for those unhealthy foods. The process does not need to be complicated or expensive as you may think.

GOOD FOOD V BAD FOOD

GOOD FOOD

Living foods or raw foods

Food that is alive is crude food. There has been no cooking, bubbling, stewing, microwave cooking, freezing, baking, or steaming of these food varieties. Hence, they actually hold their food catalysts and are in their unique state. The chemicals in food assume a significant part in processing. Growing grains, grew seeds, crude natural products, and crude vegetables all contain food catalysts. To keep a solid digestion and sustain our bodies, we require an overflow of food proteins.

The weight control plans of members in You Is What You Eat were generally underhanded on the grounds that they had no food chemicals. Most of members had eaten nothing crude.

Great carbs

A starch without refined sugar is one that contains organic product, entire grain, grains, rice, and vegetables without added sugar. Normal sugars tracked down in these mind boggling carbs (called complex carbs) assist the body with directing its temperament, energy levels, and cerebrum capability.
They are not deprived of their supplements.

Natural food varieties

The term natural alludes to food varieties that are without synthetic. Agrochemicals and pesticides have not been utilized to prepare or shower natural harvests. It is essential to remember that poisonous synthetics will enter your body assuming they have been showered on the item you eat from synthetically treated soil. Is it conceivable to foresee the harm they will cause? A few investigations show that our bodies don't profit from the synthetic substances inside.

Great protein

Proteins from vegetables are effortlessly processed by the body. There are not many veggie lover proteins as simple to process as quinoa. Porridge can be made with it, and it seems to be a grain. The fledglings we eat (not Brussels sprouts, yet seeds developed from seeds) are more reasonable, better, and more proficient than meat. It is not difficult to process and improves the digestion when beans and grains are consolidated together, bringing about a total protein.

Great fats

It's obviously true that fats are awful for you. Without fat eating regimens and low-fat food have nearly transformed the campaign against fats into franticness. Avocados can never be faulted for coronary illness, even by the most passionate campaigners!
My patients frequently get some information about nuts, seeds, and avocados, which are great fat food varieties. It is essential to eat oil-rich food varieties since they contain solid fats, which help weight reduction, lower cholesterol, upgrade invulnerability, feed regenerative organs, skin, hair, and bone tissue, and successfully grease up the body.
Great fats are crucial forever and vital for endurance. You can use fat all the more proficiently with these fats. Since they are so vital, they are alluded to as fundamental unsaturated fats (EFAs).
EFAs can't be created by the body, so you should eat them through food. Fundamental Thinny

Acids would be a superior name for them. The small idea appears to speak to my patients more than the huge idea in my training. The absolute best wellsprings of fundamental, metallic fats are flax seeds, sunflower seeds, pumpkin seeds, ocean vegetables, and avocados.
We are nearly a fat campaign gone frantic.

Natural food varieties

Synthetics or different added substances are not added to these food sources. The food is as it was developed essentially, in its unique state. No progressions have been made. Food sources fixings actually stay in their unique state in a few bundled food varieties. Investigate the marks on the food you eat and get familiar with what goes into them.

Terrible FOOD

Terrible carbs

Starches that are basic are sweet and refined. A couple of models incorporate chocolates, cakes, bread rolls, and desserts made with refined sugars and faded white rice. Subsequent to refining, most of nutrients and minerals are eliminated from the food, so it acts like sugar when it enters the body. Accordingly, blood glucose levels are upset, and sugar desires happen. You will without a doubt encounter state of mind swings in the event that you devour an excessive number of these food varieties. Discouragement, outrage, and crabbiness might happen. The most ideal way to put on weight and become sick is to eat terrible carbs. Fat is put away in the body when terrible carb deposits are exorbitant. It is likewise conceivable to foster diabetes following quite a while of consuming terrible carbs. It is a waste of time to face the challenge.

Non-natural food varieties

Synthetic manures and pesticides are utilized to treat non-natural soil and develop non-natural leafy foods. These synthetic compounds are found in non-natural food varieties, which are then consumed into our bodies. Our stomach related frameworks and cells are harmed by them. Our bodies become harmed and dirtied by these synthetic substances.

Terrible protein

There are sure proteins that might be inadequate for you relying upon the strength of your stomach related framework. In For getting healthy, the kind of food you eat is everything, most members had an extremely feeble stomach related framework, so red meat proteins were difficult to process.

Creature food varieties high in protein, fat, and red can toxify the body, add to the fermentation of the blood, drain calcium, over-burden the kidneys and the liver, smother processing, and annihilate great microorganisms in the stomach. Other than causing kidney stones and liver weariness, this may likewise prompt colon and inside problems, blockage, joint inflammation, osteoporosis, and cardiovascular infection.

There are many individuals who experience issues processing even cow's milk. Beside sinusitis, asthma, ear infections, clog, runny noses, skin rashes, dermatitis, weariness, dormancy, and touchiness, it can likewise set off hypersensitive reactions. In spite of its high immersed fat substance, low nutrient substance, and out-of-balance mineral substance, entire cow's milk can't assimilate numerous supplements by people. The milk of cows is additionally frequently defiled by many various medications, chemicals, pesticides, and buildups of these substances. To make cow's milk more straightforward to process, bubble it first.

On the other hand, goat's and sheep's milk are more straightforward to separate because of their more modest atoms. Moreover, there are some simple to-process sorts of milk available: rice milks, soy milks, and different grains.

Refined food varieties

The cutting edge diet contains many refined food varieties. Every one of the members on Your health will depend on the type of food you eat had consumes less calories brimming with refined food sources. Refined food sources are deprived of their unique, normal supplement content and fiber. The customer is left with a more focused, unnatural sweet form of the first food. Refined endlessly white sugar are the two most normal instances of refined food varieties. These fixings are then utilized in a huge number of other 'food varieties.' Heated products, chocolates, quick food varieties, and prepared dinners, to give some examples, have a more extended time span of usability; these food varieties contain added substances and additives. These food varieties truly ought to be called 'non-food varieties.' They cause devastation with the strength of the body as the body isn't intended to manage this supplement

Drained, modern, misleading food sources. On the show, I met one member who just ate refined, handled, additive loaded food sources. Yvonne, who was overweight, discouraged, depleted, and obstructed, endure basically on crisps and microwaved dinners. She never under any circumstance ate genuine food. To carry Yvonne to her detects, I teasingly recommended that if she somehow managed to drop dead tomorrow, her body would in a real sense require a very long time to disintegrate on the grounds that she was so brimming with this large number of additives. The message most certainly overcame, notwithstanding the shock! ... long stretches of terrible carb eating could prompt diabetes. It's not worth the gamble.

Awful fats

Immersed creature fats are weighty and go to stone inside the body, solidifying the courses and leaving you in danger of coronary failure and stroke. Red meat, pork, dairy items, margarine, and cheddar are instances of food sources that are fat-soaked. The body isn't intended to manage these kinds of fats. High terrible fat eating regimens raise circulatory strain and cholesterol levels, can disrupt glucose levels, and cause liver stagnation, which can prompt sorrow and weight gain. The body can't successfully deal with awful fats, so many are transformed into harmful balls and put away in the body, making you much fatter. Hydrogenated fats are the consequences of a cycle that solidifies fluid vegetable oils. Shortening and margarine are hydrogenated fats, so potato chips, chocolate, desserts, frozen yogurt, cakes, and prepared merchandise all contain hydrogenated fats. The hydrogenated fats change into evermore perilous trans-unsaturated fats, which have been displayed to cause diabetes, coronary illness, and malignant growth.
Trans unsaturated fats additionally make you put on weight as they disrupt the digestion and

breakdown of fundamental unsaturated fats. They increment the terrible cholesterol in the body and exhaust the upside.

Handled food sources

The handling of food sources changes the first food and the extents of the supplements inside these food sources. Numerous pre-bundled and plastic-wrapped food sources, speedy x, microwaveable, quick, and heating up the-sack type food sources, have gone through a large number of cycles before they end up in the store. These food sources have next to zero healthy benefit. The food business permits in excess of 3000 food added substances to be utilized

In the handling of food. Also, on the grounds that a considerable lot of these added substances and synthetics utilized in the handling of our food sources are considered safe, it doesn't imply that they are. Thus, synthetics, food added substances, shading specialists, sugars, counterfeit flavors, colors, nitrates, nitrites, additives to forestall deterioration, acids, developing, fading specialists, and emulsifiers to keep up with consistency are finding their direction into our bodies by means of these simple to-get ready bundled food sources. These cycles can make hypersensitive responses weight on the liver to handle such synthetics, a large number of which are disease shaping.
Kids presented to such cycles can become hyperactive and show learning hardships.

Eating better is somewhat more costly, however it brings down your gamble of sickness, which brings down your medical services costs, which are a lot higher than good dieting.

FOCUS ON YOU

In the end, your weight loss success is determined by how you feel about yourself. Physical concerns are the most important thing to most people. They didn't know that an obvious result didn't start from the outside. It started way long in my mind. And that is why this is part of my tricks to losing weight fast. Focus on you yourself!

Reducing extra pounds is the problem, perhaps, of most men and women who requires a lot of work, courage, patience, and willpower. But often, the hours spent on the simulator, strenuous exercises, and exhausting hunger strikes do not give the desired result; weight loss does not occur. But many people do not even realize that you can lose weight using a simple and enjoyable way. This slimming meditation is asimple and natural tool that will help promote progress in weight loss.

Meditation is often seen as a relaxing practice, but one that benefits the mind only, not the body. Indeed, when you think, "I have to lose weight," you will tend to see yourself exercising more and dieting. However, the first step in these two methods isbasically going through your head. So, we will see how we can effectively practice meditation to lose weight.

HOW MEDITATION HELPS LOSE WEIGHT

It would seem that how meditation can help you lose weight. But in fact, meditationpractice has many advantages:

Metabolism regulation. With regular practice, the human body restores its biological functions, including metabolism. This contributes to the fact that weightloss occurs naturally, and fat deposits go away. A good metabolism in the body also causes a decrease in appetite, which is why a person eats less.

Digestion. Meditation helps to improve the absorption of food. Hormonal imbalances in the female body and stress lead to overeating and indigestion. Regularexercise helps relax your nerves and balance hormones. This has a long-term impacton efforts to reduce extra pounds.

Legibleness in food. One of the best deterrents to weight reduction is the desire for undesirable and unfortunate food sources. Thinning reflection wipes out these undesirable desires. An individual turns out to be more mindful of what he eats, as he deals with his own body and in this way sheds pounds.

Stress opposition. All the time, indulging happens because of stress. Encountering, an individual himself doesn't see the development of his hunger. This prompts a bunch of additional pounds. For that reason contemplation is fundamental for shedding pounds since it kills the essential wellspring of the issue — it diminishes pressure.

Discipline. Uncontrolled dinners and bites are related with the way that an individual can't decline his number one food. The best way flawlessly is confidence in oneself, resolve, lucidity of psyche, and discipline. By thinking consistently, this large number of characteristics can be created and fortified oneself.

Self-spellbinding. A lot is had some significant awareness of the force of thought — they emerge and turn into a reality on the off chance that endeavors are made. For this situation, contemplation works like spellbinding — an individual projects himself for the outcome.

Instructions to Get thinner WHILE Contemplating

Contemplation on concordance ought to be an everyday practice. For adequacy, thinking day to day for somewhere around 20 minutes is suggested.

Thinning contemplation doesn't need to be troublesome. In the event that you're a fledgling, take a stab at beginning five minutes in the first part of the day to clear your psyche prior to facing a bustling day and five minutes prior to hitting the sack. Yoga teachers note that, on a basic level, the hour of classes doesn't make any difference on the off chance that you contemplate consistently and accurately. As per surveys, you can see the consequences of getting in shape provided that reflection turns into a propensity.

The standards of contemplation if you have any desire to get more fit

Utilize a mantra to assist you with getting in shape. A mantra is a platitude or maxim that you rehash to yourself to zero in on the objective when your psyche meanders. These are words that can ultimately go into reflective spellbinding.

Watch your breath. Do whatever it takes not to change your breathing as you shut your eyes. Assuming your brain meanders — and it will be so right away — simply direct it back to your breath.

Reflection for greatness in getting thinner ought not be unpleasant. Simultaneously, an individual ought to feel good, and this applies to everything: Dress, pose, climate, prosperity

Bit by bit Guidance

Any individual who needs to get in shape can think. To work out, there is no requirement for extraordinary hardware or costly classes. For some, the hardest part is carving out the opportunity to do as such. Yet, headed straight toward your objective, you can make it happen.

Ensure you have the chance to make quiet for the time you want.

At the point when you end up in a peaceful spot, quiet yourself and unwind. You can rests in any advantageous position.

Begin by zeroing in on your breath, noticing your chest or stomach when it rises and falls. Feel the air as it moves and leaves your mouth or nose. Pay attention to the sounds that the air makes. Do this briefly until you start to feel more loose.

Then, with your eyes open or shut, do the accompanying: Take a full breath. Hold it for a couple of moments. Breathe out leisurely and rehash. Breathe in normally. Notice your breathing when it enters your noses, raises your chest, or moves to your stomach, however keep it that way. Continue to zero in on your breath for 5-10 minutes.

Begin to picture. Envision how you are thin and lovely, put on your number one dress, how you stroll along the catwalk, how men pivot after you. In weight reduction reflection, ladies must build their confidence to comprehend that change is fundamental for their flawlessness of themselves.

Contemplation RESULTS IN Weight reduction

To contemplate explicitly to shed pounds, search for practices zeroed in on this. Getting thinner contemplation seems to be entrancing or self-spellbinding. Shaping the force of thought, the force of will is significant. It is vital to present for yourself that you truly need something (to get more fit in this present circumstance) and endeavor to satisfy your longing. This can be a perception of how you can look and feel after you have shed pounds. You can envision yourself thin and thin, intellectually getting into your #1 garments.

Yet, with every one of the advantages of reflection while getting more fit, it is just a single strategy in a bunch of activities for shedding pounds. It is difficult to shed pounds by simply pondering. Assuming you eat kilograms of chips and buns and can't lessen your craving, then, at that point, even numerous long stretches of reflection won't save you and won't assist with diminishing weight.

Legitimate sustenance and exercise are likewise significant pieces of the way to agreement. There will constantly be improved outcomes on the off chance that you join this multitude of parts into one and make them your lifestyle.

First of all, reflective practice changes the reasoning, awareness, and demeanor to the issue and assists with reinforcing endlessly longing for the objective. Concentrates on show that these progressions require just 21 days. It is in three weeks that an individual's propensities change and structure, including eating right and eating pretty much nothing, denying low quality food, and drinking a lot of water — this likewise assists with getting thinner.

Reflection has noteworthy power since we partner feelings coming from the profundities of the spirit with cognizant idea. In reflection, the individual is brought into a similar recurrence as the beginning of the Internal identity, or at least, the actual Universe, and in this way is straightforwardly associated with the cognizance circle of the Universe. In this state, there is no time limit, so the pictured satisfaction can quickly extend to the actual level. Because of customary contemplation, we get various advantages in a physical and mental sense.

We will be better since when we center around our breathing, our circulatory strain drops, and our pulse dials back; subsequently, we become more settled. It assists us with having a more clear brain to figure out our viewpoints and feelings, making our correspondence more useful both at work and in public activity. We can concentrate all the more effectively and in like manner feel less anxious. We become more mindful of our feelings; consequently, we can oversee them all the more actually. We find an answer sooner in parts of our lives where we feel stuck. It advances the handling of mental issues. It assists with discovering a true sense of harmony and equilibrium.

TECHNIQUE OF MEDITATION

Conscious Meditation

It's easy to get hooked up in a loop of spinning thoughts — starting to think about alaundry list of activities to do, ruminating about past events, or potentially future situations — and practicing mindfulness may help. Yet, what exactly is attention? Mentally, mindfulness involves focusing on the present moment without judging what you are thinking, feeling, or sensing.

Mindfulness meditation is a form of mental preparation that helps you to slow downthoughts of running, let go of anger, and relax both your mind and body. Mindfulness methods can vary, but a meditation on mindfulness generally involves breathing exercises, mental imagery, body and mind awareness, and relaxation of the muscle and organs. Practicing meditation with mindfulness does not require props or planning (no need for candles, essential oils, or mantras, unless you enjoy it). All youneed is a comfortable sitting spot, three to five minutes of spare time, and an attitudethat's free of judgment.

Mindfulness meditation is the method of having your thoughts fully present. Knowledge involves being mindful of where we are and what we do and not being toosensitive to what is happening around us.

One can do reflective meditation anywhere. Some people like to relax in a quiet spot,close their eyes, and focus on their respiration. But at every stage of the day, even when driving to work or doing chores, you can choose to be conscious.

You track your thoughts and feelings while practicing mindfulness meditation but letthem move without judgment.

Transcendental meditation: Transcendental meditation is an essential techniquewhereby an individually defined rhythm, such as a word, sound, or short phrase, is repeated in a particular way. It is exercised twice per day for 20 minutes while sittingcomfortably close to the eyes.

The hope is that this technique will allow you to settle into a deep state of relaxationto achieve inner peace without attention or effort.

Directed Meditation:

Coordinated contemplation, frequently likewise alluded to as directed symbolism or perception, is a reflection method wherein you make mental pictures or situations that you track down quieting.

Directed contemplation is among the most widely recognized strategies for reflection utilized consistently by a large number of individuals. Here, we'll investigate directed reflection and how to make it happen.

In the most perfect structure, directed reflection is a kind of contemplation where the individual is directed on each step of his everyday practice. Somebody guides you right from the primary degree of sitting in a reflective posture to the last period of finishing the contemplation. What happens is that during contemplation, an instructor or coach gives bit by bit direction about what to do. It is an old technique for passing headings for contemplation on to understudies. In more seasoned times, this procedure was utilized to show reflection in a gathering. These days, because of mechanical turn of events, we never again need a master's actual presence to lead us in reflection. We can pay attention to an expert's immediate direction utilizing pre-recorded Discs or DVDs and lead our contemplation practice. Without any reflection ace proficient Discs/DVDs, you can record the

Directions of directed reflection from a book in your voice and afterward play them a while later.

Moreover, on the off chance that anybody doesn't have the capacity of a voice recorder or a blue ray player, during a meeting, he might ask his companions or family members to orally talk the composed contemplation guidelines. Along these lines, we can utilize the advantage of directed reflection with next to no innovative help.

In any case, I actually accept that the utilization of a pre-recorded Compact disc or DVD for directed reflection is the most effective way for directed contemplation, as it eliminates the requirement for an individual to be truly present close to you to peruse the guidelines. It additionally allows you to exploit controlled contemplation, in any event, when you're distant from everyone else.

Directed guidelines for contemplation can be of different assortments relying upon the strategies the instructor confers. Probably the most widely recognized reflection methods utilized in directed contemplation are Vipassana - which includes representation of the pattern of breathing, visual creative mind, mantra recitation, a reflection on moving, a reflection on supplication, a contemplation on care, and so forth. The least demanding method for utilizing directed contemplation is to pay attention to an expert's live direction. In the event that this isn't achievable, then, at that point, the second-most ideal choice is to keep in your voice the composed guidelines of contemplation and afterward stand by listening to them in your reflection practice.

Normally, this stage is coordinated by an aide or educator, hence "determined." It is likewise recommended that you use however many faculties as could be expected under the circumstances, like fragrance, sounds, and surfaces, to evoke tranquility in your loosening up district.

Vipassana Contemplation: Vipassana reflection is an old type of Indian reflection, and that implies seeing things as they are. Over a long time back, it was shown in India. The cognizant reflection development has starting points in this training in the US.

The motivation behind contemplation with vipassana is self-change through the assessment of oneself. This is achieved to make a profound association among brain and body via cautious consideration regarding the sensations in the body. The supported interconnectedness prompts a blissful record loaded up with adoration and empathy.

Vipassana is normally educated during a 10-day course in this custom, and individuals are supposed to observe a bunch of guidelines constantly, as well as going without all intoxicants, lying, cheating, sexual action, and killing any creatures.

Cherishing contemplation on empathy (metta reflection): Metta contemplation, additionally called reflection on adoring benevolence, is the act of directing great wishes towards others. The people who work on recounting comparative words and expressions will inspire caring opinions. This is likewise usually tracked down in reflection on care and vipassana.

It's typically finished in a wonderful, loosened up position while sitting. After a couple of full breaths, you gradually and consistently rehash the accompanying words. "Just let me be cheerful. May I be fine? Allow me to be free. May I be quiet and calm." After a time of directing this cherishing generosity to yourself, you might start to envision a relative or companion who has upheld you and rehash the mantra, this time supplanting "I" with "you." As you proceed with the reflection, you might infer different individuals from your family, companions, neighbors, or individuals in your day to day existence. Professionals are frequently urged to consider people who are experiencing difficulty with them.

At long last, you finish the contemplation with the standard mantra: "Let each being be cheerful all over" — a reflection on the Chakra.

Chakra is an old Sanskrit term that can be followed back to India and converts into a "cycle." The chakras allude to the energy and profound power habitats inside the

Body. It is accepted there will be seven chakras. Each chakra is in an alternate piece of the body, and every one of them has a comparing tone.

Chakra reflection comprises of unwinding methods that mean to carry cquilibrium and prosperity to the chakras. Any of these strategies gives the visual portrayal of any chakra in the body and the relating light. Certain individuals can like to light incense or use gems, which are variety coded for each Chakra to assist them with centering during reflection.

Reflection yoga: The yoga practice has its underlying foundations in old India. There is a wide assortment of yoga classes and styles, however all incorporate playing out a progression of stances and directed breathing activities intended to empower adaptability and loosen up the psyche.

The stances require equilibrium and consideration, and specialists are urged to focus less on interruptions and stay more at the time.

Which reflection style you decide to attempt relies upon a few elements. At the point when you have a medical condition and are new to yoga, let your PCP know what technique might really work out for you.

Contemplation AND Weight reduction

Supernatural Contemplation and Weight reduction

Contemplation is by and large used as a loosening up instrument, like a back rub for the mind. In addition, similarly as there are various ways to deal with making a natural item serving of leafy greens, contemplation goes with an arrangement of frameworks. One explicit sort called Supernatural Contemplation (TM) has procured the differentiation since the 1960s after a commended melodic team called "The Beatles" started practicing it.

TM isn't a religion, thinking, or lifestyle. Rather, it is a method for achieving a more conspicuous sensation of congruity and calm in day to day existence, likewise the benefit of being accessible. Whether or not you are searching for more unmistakable significance all through daily existence, searching for lightening from anxiety, or wanting to prevent fast thoughts, reflection might help. It is sensible to see that every one of the as of late referred to reasons unbelievably affect our general prosperity and, progressively, our weight.

The essential difference that isolates supernatural contemplation and various kinds of strategies is the mantra approach during a reflection meeting. The mantra is contrasted with a vehicle, which is being utilized to assist the brain with tracking down a quiet spot and settle down.

It is the most normal and simple arrangement of contemplation. In any case, it is similarly the most evolved and, from an overall perspective, unmistakable system considering the way that the ease relies upon a critical and complete understanding of the cerebrum and its direct as well as the body, and how the two connection point during significant reflection, something not grasped in every practical sense, as a few different techniques. Along these lines, a constraint of 20 minutes, two times each day, sitting in a pleasing seat are together that is required.

Here are the resources to practice TM:

- Sit down, expecting an agreeable position. Try not to fold your arms or legs.

- Ensure your eyes are shut. Take a few full breaths to bring the body into unwinding.

- Wake up and close them again. Your eyes will accept this state for the entire 20-minute span.

- Settle on the mantra to discuss to you.

- At the point when you notice that the psyche has begun to meander, pull together your consideration back on the mantra.

- After the entire term is finished, gradually move your toes and fingers to get yourself once again to the real world.

- Wake up.

- On the off chance that you don't feel ready to happen with your day, sit for a more drawn out term.

To be sure, you could contemplate how TM will assist with weight decline. According to research directed at veterans experiencing PTSD, when the psyche rises above, the body comes into an expression that is far more profound than even profound rest and goes there undeniably more rapidly. Stress prompts a characteristic instrument,which is intended for our assurance to endure. This pressure logically triggers various exercises to counter the response:

- The front piece of the cerebrum will be detached, the part which is liable for drivecontrol.
- The creation of the bliss hormone "dopamine" diminishes (the pressure hormone"cortisol" increments.
- Individuals under pressure are less and less able to tune in to the normal needs of thebody.

Rising above is fundamentally the contrary experience of pressure, and that way, it will have contrary impacts. The subsequent harmony enables the body to likewise increase exceptionally profound rest (further than rest), in which it can disintegrate even its most profound anxieties aggregated because of life's most exceedingly terrible injuries. As we develop, revive, and renew from the quietness of meditation, this can possibly, deliver different emotional upgrades in any part of ourlife.

As you can see, meditation is the key to harmony, an amazing technique in which there is not a single side effect. This practice can change a person, both internally andphysically, for the better.

CREATE YOUR NEW LIFESTYLE

The utilization of lifestyle changes and behavioral modification to manage weight is based on the body of evidence that suggests that people get or are overweight as a result of alterable behavior or habits and that, through changing these behaviors, theweight will be reduced and sustained.

You must continue to modify your lifestyle in order to maintain weight loss. In the long run, you will gain weight if you return to the habits that led to your weight gain. A healthy eating and exercise routine is imperative to permanently lose weight, just as you developed them during the weight loss process. The majority of people who lose weight gain it back right after they relax their vigilance too much. Having reached your goal, you can relax a little -- but not too much.

ALL ABOUT A HEALTHY LIFESTYLE

For you, the word "healthy lifestyle" could mean a boring lifestyle that is brimming with juice from carrots. But this isn't an accurate definition. Being mindful of your body's health as the primary goal in your life is not as difficult as some might think, asit can help your life be more enjoyable. Life is enjoyable, and you'd prefer not to be stifled by useless health problems. Today, your organs of vital importance (kidney, digestive tracts, kidneys, ink bladder, heart, stomach, liver, lungs, etc., Obesity-related) might be functioning superbly. But they might not be in the near future.

Don't overestimate your good health now. Be sure to take well to take care of yourself. Achieving great health isn't only about healthy eating habits and physical activity but also about maintaining positive mental health and a positive self-image,and a balanced lifestyle. A long, stressful feeling of joy awaits you in these steps on the off chance you're doing it correctly. Healthier living is within your reach. Start itnow. It is evident that being healthy is in line with the direction of duty.

IMPORTANCE OF A HEALTHY LIFESTYLE

It is critical to comprehend that the significance of carrying on with a sound life isn't just about the actual viewpoint, nonetheless. Albeit by and large, residing sound propensities in our homes is really great for us truly, it likewise decidedly affects each and every part of our lives. The upsides of a solid way of life are:

- Dispensing with or decreasing ongoing ailments, for example, hypertension, diabetes, heart weight-related sicknesses

- Characterizing the dangers of profound shakiness

- Developing degrees of imperativeness

- Upgrading sexual limit and mystique

The meaning of carrying on with a solid way of life is recognized in different viewpoints that we live. At the point when we take care to work on our physical and psychological wellness and advantage soundly and truly, proceeding to carry on with a better way of life permits us to make a more inspirational outlook. At the point when we feel more joyful and great, we have positive expectations about ourselves. What's more, as trust in ourselves and certainty increments, we notice an improvement in our collaborations with others. Individuals will quite often be attracted to individuals with positive characteristics about themselves, and having prosperity and a sound way of life will definitely help us in becoming somebody who others need to spend time with. It's gainful to our lives as people, yet it can help our expert lives too.

Assuming we take a gander at what solid living could mean for our lives, obviously disregarding the significance of a sound and adjusted lifestyle is beyond the realm of possibilities. Yet, as you can envision, solid living goes substantially more than simply improving our eating regimen routine and adding a touch of wellness to our step by step daily schedule. Making changes to our old propensities requires commitment and exertion, yet likewise the case it's conceivable it's surely smart disregarding all the problem.

Advantages TO A Solid Lifestyle

With the better comprehension of our bodies, which we've gained from science during the most recent couple of many years, The advantages of carrying on with a sound life are accompanying a more clear picture and the reasoning behind for us to scrub our body consistently to check for hurtful microorganisms, even the worms that occupy our stomach-related structure. For all ages, limits, loads, and sizes, the advantages of a fair way of life are perpetual. Meanwhile, imagine a scenario in which we check out at eight basic advantages of a functioning way of life.

1. Your Wellbeing:

Great wellbeing isn't something you can purchase at a medication shop or retail foundation however can be accomplished by learning the most well-known wellbeing related ways of behaving with regards to the accessible choices. In accordance with this rationale, if you're hoping to become familiar with the upsides of a sound way of life, evaluating a genuine model in your week after week exercises is fundamental. There are numerous instances of practicing good eating habits and working out. Benefits incorporate Reduced medical care costs, less disease and wounds, less visits to trained professionals, keeping you utilized, and further developed business/laborer connections.

2. Weight:

Monitoring how much weight you convey is the way to partaking in the best piece of the relative multitude of advantages related with a solid way of life. A weight reduction of 10% will essentially diminish the possibility experiencing coronary illnesses and other medical problems connected with power.
Heaviness/overweight is the subsequent driving contributing part to various young adult infections, for instance, muscular dissipates, rest apnea, sort II diabetes mellitus, asthma, hypertension and cholesterol, skin issue, excited and psychosocial issues (Spigel, 2002), and impressive more. Practice that is weight-bearing, like strolling, walking, and strength preparing, can slow the advancement of osteoporosis, and some exploration proposes that partaking in such exercises can fabricate bone mass and start to switch the impacts of

The sickness. Different advantages incorporate weight decrease pressure, diminished strain, and tension, worked on prosperity, worked on mental self portrait and confidence, as well as a supported actual capacity.

3. Exercise:

Regardless of the way that prescription alone will frequently lessen cholesterol back to typical, a sound eating regimen routine and exercise can give benefits that drugs can't.

They can diminish the burden on the circulatory framework as well as lessen weight and decrease the gamble of creating diabetes. This sickness can be exacerbated by a way of life is latent. Customary activity and a sound eating regimen routine will assist the body with utilizing insulin all the more successfully and will support diminishing, controlling, and forestalling the improvement of numerous infections. Work out, quit smoking utilization, the right eating regimen, which is a low-fat and high-fiber program, lessen body weight, and comprehend how to conform to extend and decrease the possibility experiencing coronary sicknesses.

4. Medical:

Everybody should be managed and have the best body wellbeing for different flavorful social, clinical and social reasons. Fortifying living is genuinely the best drug. In a review drove by Tufts School at the New England Clinical Center on individuals experiencing cardiovascular illness, the work-out routine was displayed to diminish LDL cholesterol in a complete way too. Another peril is that it goes past what's given by the drug. Indeed, even unpretentious weight issues can support diminishing the expense of clinical and drug store and assist with staying away from bariatric medical procedure as well as co-morbidities like hypertension, asthma, and diabetes.

5. Wellness:

Being agreeable inside your own space, your body, your disposition, and your state. An even way of life can decisively broaden the life expectancy of a man. Also, despite the fact that getting this season's virus or cold isn't many times a chance knowing that having a solid tendency is an optimal lifestyle choice ought to provoke them to scrutinize the explanation you're not trying to carry on with their life in the most effective way that could be conceivable under the current conditions. The issue with a many individuals today is that they're so participated in taking care of their business as well as managing the world in their lives that they disregard their wellbeing and prosperity. Ensure you have a solid heart healthy, and your bones serious areas of strength for are, keep on following that way to receive the rewards of a reasonable way of life.

6. Care:

The most effective way to guarantee great wellbeing is to manage your own wellbeing. A ton of your medical services is in question; nonetheless, the advantages are gigantic in forestalling unexpected passing or a silly disease handicap, diminishing the wellbeing medical services costs, and guaranteeing that you keep the best quality of living into advanced age. Assuming that you carry on with a sound way of life is your own character, and you're not expected to be aware of what ordinarily would cause you to feel if you could think often much about your life.

7. Control:

On the off chance that you carry on with a sound and adjusted way of life, it is simpler for you to control your predetermination since you battle your body to ward off those parts of life that might attempt to cause you to feel down in the impossible occasion that you permit them to. On the off chance that you have the advantages of a better way of life, you can take the capacity to control your rest examples, and you will feel rested over the course of your day. At the point when you carry on with a solid way of life, it is feasible for all that to make various parts of your day to day routine, and it will help you. The logical proof has shown that the impacts of solid weight and good dieting propensities and wellbeing plans can bring about astonishing enhancements in wellbeing and help in forestalling normal illnesses like elevated cholesterol and circulatory strain, diabetes, hypertension, stress, and general absence of energy.

8. Strength:

One more benefit of a solid way of life is a consistent progression of solidarity and endurance. You can perform exercises as well as activities that work on your fitness. At the point when you carry on with a solid and adjusted way of life, you have modified and unmistakable restraint from food sources that give your body the vital supplements and energy. You're sufficiently able to assemble the muscles that help joints and bones; by doing this, you lessen the gamble of falling and cracks. Practice that is cardiovascular, or oxygen-consuming activities, further develop the heart muscle and, along these lines, builds the productivity of the heart. The weight and strength of our bones normally decline as we age.

Practice that is weight-bearing, like strolling, strolling, and reinforcing, can slow the movement of osteoporosis and some exploration recommends that a sharp excitement for these exercises can increment bone thickness and start to invert the impacts of osteoporosis.

As a matter of fact, you don't have to prepare to be an Olympic member to partake in every one of the benefits related with a better way of life. The secret and the thinking are rehashing a picked customary model that can be utilized as a component of your everyday or week-by-week exercises. We are certain that this will assist you with accomplishing the place of a better life in the impossible occasion that you're not yet there. A solid life is a lifestyle.

Careful discipline brings about promising results

You become better at something as you practice it. Making solid propensities a piece of your everyday schedule takes time. As opposed to allowing all your persistent effort to go to squander, show restraint toward yourself. Arrangement is vital to knowing your shortcomings. Allurements will emerge when you devour specific food varieties and in specific conditions, however following your determination will assist you with defeating them. When confronted with troublesome conditions, control is the best methodology.

To keep a solid weight, I in some cases permit myself a little extravagance on one day of the week. There is no week-to-week minor departure from this day;

Try not to allow this valuable chance to cruise you by, and you could end up requiring over one day "off" each week because of conditions. During the assigned free day, which for me is Saturday, I permit myself to enjoy my #1 food sources for however long they are sensibly speaking. You needn't bother with the whole cheesecake, simply a little piece! Essentially, it's deceiving taken care of.

SUCCESSFUL LOSERS

The people who have prevailed in weight reduction can furnish us with some knowledge.

Individuals who have lost or kept up with something like 60 pounds for at least five years are followed by the Public Weight Control Library (NWCR). Their exercises include:

Record it on paper. You can keep yourself on target by journaling your food admission.

Eat light and right. Low-fat weight control plans work the best for best failures since extraordinary eating regimen food sources, wizardry pills, and contrivances aren't economical. Work-out day to day. Like cleaning their teeth, strolling is a must-do movement for these individuals. Around one hour of activity is done consistently by NWCR individuals.
Begin the day with breakfast. Sound mornings are upheld by all exploration.
Show up consistently. Returning to their sound weight is their prompt need in the event that they gain a couple of pounds.
Keeping the load off for a significant stretch of time makes it more straightforward to keep up with the misfortune. Fruitful washouts track down satisfaction in their new ways of life, and carrying on with a better life no longer feels like an errand. The objective ought to be to carry on with a sound way of life, not to count calories. Over the long haul, keeping up with weight becomes more straightforward. Nearly every individual who arrives at the two-year point is brilliant.

Continue through to the end

Keep your inspiration high and don't allow difficulties to get you off course: Assuming that you tumble off the cart, simply dismiss yourself and return to your triumphant ways. In the event that you can figure out how to take on a similar mindset as a slight individual and act in like manner, you'll remain slender until the end of time. Also, the more you practice, the simpler it becomes. When you get to the upkeep level, odds are you have distinguished examples, methods, and abilities that have ended up being useful in keeping you on target.

Reward yourself. You ought to be praised for rolling out solid improvements in your eating regimen and work-out schedules that not just act as a motivation to your loved ones yet in addition have colossal medical advantages

Research has shown that staying in touch with individuals or projects (like WebMD's Weight reduction Facility) that assist you with getting in shape is connected to long haul weight upkeep. It's a good idea to remain associated with individuals who assisted you with prevailing in any case. So keep close by and let us assist you with keeping up with your weight reduction!

Put forth Objectives

Defining objectives to shed pounds is fundamental for a solid, success. The most common way of defining objectives might show up simple beyond a shadow of a doubt. Others may be in a tight spot when they attempt to sort out some way to put forth objectives. Laying out objectives should be thoroughly examined and practical, or you could subvert your weight reduction endeavors. On the off chance that you make a rash objective, your ability to stay engaged and persuaded is hampered right all along.

The objective is to make an arrangement to change your way of life in the progress to a better day to day daily schedule. The objectives you set need to assist you with diminishing your weight as well as work on your general wellbeing. What could shock you is that the initial step while making an arrangement is to decide if you genuinely require weight reduction and if talking with a specialist could be the most ideal choice. At the point when you, alongside your primary care physician, establish that weight decrease is a need, this is the ideal opportunity to begin making your objective!

Process Versus Result Objectives

Objectives for weight reduction can be characterized into two gatherings - result objectives and cycle goals. To make your weight reduction plan viable, you'll require both. You're making progress toward an objective for the final product. For example, it very well may be the weight you might want to lose. Result based objectives can assist you with concentrating. Nonetheless, they don't give strategies to arrive.

Process objectives characterize what you should be aware, the "how" of accomplishing your ideal weight reduction result, and furnish you with a technique to stick to. Instances of weight reduction objectives for the cycle incorporate strolling for 30 minutes every day, staying away from pastries at dinnertime, or subbing drinks with water. These objectives can be more significant than objective situated results since they modify your way of life to empower weight reduction.

The most important phase in laying out your objectives is to figure out the two kinds, and you should comply to the rules for weight reduction objectives. This implies the result and objectives should be explicit and quantifiable.

Put forth Savvy objectives for weight reduction

A Savvy objective is:

- Explicit
- Quantifiable
- Feasible
- Significant
- Time-delicate

Objectives for weight reduction

It is feasible to start by examining these parts of your eating regimen methodology with your doctor. They will actually want to give master guidance and data that can help you in defining your cycle and result objectives. There are different assets to contemplate in view of your particular targets.

Explicit

The objective should be explicit and exact. A many individuals put forth out determined to get fit. It is an overall objective and doesn't have a particular goal. What's the significance here for you to become better? Eating better? Would you like to eliminate liquor and nicotine? What are your choices for handling this goal?

A superior objective incorporates explicit subtleties. For example, an objective to eat better isn't explicit. Notwithstanding, a goal to kill sweets, quit drinking soda pops that are sweet, and have something like 1 or two foods grown from the ground at each feast is unmistakable. You've pursued a choice on the moves you'll make and when you'll finish them.

We should define a Shrewd objective for weight reduction today. In lieu of the standard thing "I need to get more fit," all that model could be "I will shed 20 pounds in four months." Presently you have an unmistakable ultimate objective, and you can lay out the circumstances to decide how you'll get in shape and the sum you will lose every month. Zeroing in on the weight you need to lose can assist you with pursuing better decisions consistently.

Quantifiable

On the off chance that you can evaluate an objective, you can utilize markers to show how much you have prevailed with regards to arriving at the objective. For instance, the target of practicing all the more much of the time isn't quantifiable. The objective of going to the exercise center on Mondays, Wednesdays, and Fridays for a time of an hour can be estimated. An objective to eat less calories

It can't be measured. In any case, the point of eating under 1,500 calories daily can be followed.

Similarly, essentially putting forth an objective to shed weight is certainly not a feasible objective. To quantify weight reduction, you should incorporate a number. What is the quantity of pounds you need to lose? What number of calories will you consume? What measure of activity will you be doing? Observing your performance is significant.

Feasible

Feasible objectives are attainable weight reduction objectives you can arrive at utilizing your assets and time. For instance, in the event that you are experiencing knee gives that make running testing for your situation, running for 30 minutes daily wouldn't be a practical objective. On the off chance that you work for extended periods or are an expert, spending an hour in the exercise center consistently probably won't be reachable too.

Yet, you can turn these objectives more reachable, such as going for a stroll for thirty minutes multiple times every week, riding a supine bicycle, or swimming, which is a low-or zero-influence work out. You may likewise have the option to fit several exercises during the end of the week into 45 minutes.

With regards to shedding weight, you ought to likewise pick a figure that you can stand to lose. 50 pounds can be lost in four months, yet it very well may be a very hazardous endeavor. Assuming your objective weight is too hard to even think about coming to, it is feasible to lose the inspiration to proceed.

A powerful method for getting a feasible weight reduction sum is, regardless, a body rate that is normal. As per studies, a five to 10 percent decrease in muscle to fat ratio is plausible for most of individuals. The ideal objective could be set to lose 6 or 7 percent of muscle versus fat. Discover that figure with your PCP, and afterward separate it into sensible pieces.

Applicable

The objectives you set are appropriate and critical to you. They ought not be an objective that somebody can set for you. Think about the main things in your day to day existence right now.

Assuming that you permit yourself the space to think about the main parts of your own life, perhaps getting thinner isn't exactly one of your goals. Provided that this is true, you should decide the explanation. What is the explanation that you genuinely must get in shape now?

Knowing the justification behind your weight reduction will give you the concentration as well as the inspiration to accomplish your objectives.

At the point when weight reduction is an issue for you, counsel your doctor for exhortation. They can assist you with deciding your everyday calorie objectives corresponding to your wellbeing and weight and furthermore an activity plan.

Time-touchy

Set a cutoff time. Cutoff times can help us start and keep on working, no matter what the end last objective. When you pick your objective, set a suitable cutoff time. Your doctor might help you with setting a sensible date. For example, on the off chance that you are hoping to shed 15 pounds, put the red hearts on the schedule preceding the date you'll have to meet and set updates on your cell phone for each of your objectives simultaneously and pursue an increment of 15 pounds.

A period cutoff won't just support you, be that as it may, however it likewise helps you in excess in good shape. Assuming the ideal weight reduction rate for most of individuals is 1 to 2 weight misfortunes each week, then, at that point, put down your point in time outline as per that. For instance, "I will lose 8% of my body weight in four months."

Present moment and Long haul Objectives

Long haul objectives assist you with checking the greater in general picture out. Long haul objectives can be a phenomenal technique to move your contemplating your point from diets to making way of life changes that are sound. Nonetheless, objectives that are long haul have all the earmarks of being too hard to even consider coming to or far off to feel rousing.

This is the justification for why transient objectives are valuable. Separating your drawn out objectives into reasonable, little pieces allows you to be glad for your achievements as they happen, yet keep your eyes and spotlight on the greater objective.

Objectives for weight reduction

Assuming your definitive objective is to shed 15 pounds north of 90 days, it is feasible to break it into more modest objectives for each schedule month, for instance, seven pounds the primary month and 4 pounds every one of the accompanying two months. Weight reduction in the beginning phases is generally more quick.

One of your objectives could be to run for 30 minutes consistently. In the event that you've never run, you could possibly start by strolling for 30 minutes every day, and afterward run for 5 minutes prior to strolling for 25 minutes, and afterward continue to build the time you run versus walk time as you foster perseverance.

At the point when you are dealing with your short and long haul targets, you'll have to audit and change objectives as the need might arise to. For example, assuming that you started little however have had achievement, yet you are presently observing that three minutes of running is faster and more pleasant, you may be leaned to take on all the more a test like running 5K races. The progressions you cause will to mirror your way of life change, which is better.

Take into consideration Misfortunes

Assuming you adjust your propensities and progress along your course, you'll confront misfortunes. Difficulties are an inescapable part of life, especially during changes to your way of life. In the event that you realize that you'll encounter difficulties and plan for them too as you can, you'll be ready to devise methodologies to manage the mishaps ahead of time. Albeit this will not keep the mishap from happening (the Christmas season!) Nonetheless, you'll be ready for it, and it probably won't be as extreme a misfortune as expected.

Taking everything into account, rolling out little improvements to your way of life is essential for weight reduction. This incorporates eating a sound eating regimen and getting normal activity. In the event that you roll out these improvements, you will be headed to a better and more joyful life.

End

Indeed, we've arrived at the finish of the book. However, before you go, I might want to give you a touch of inspiration to assist you with continuing through to the end. My recommendation is straightforward: Audit the nine stunts to recognize basic moves you can initiate to obtain prompt outcomes. Yet again as a fast recap, here are the nine stunts;

- Deal with you
- Move your body
- Segment your food
- Take more leafy foods
- Feeling great is tied in with practicing good eating habits
- Plunk down and eat
- Ponder how practicing good eating habits will work on your wellbeing
- Center around yourself
- Make and adjust to your new way of life

I concede that following these straightforward tricks will be troublesome. Yet, in the event that you center around little wins and accomplishing basic objectives over the course of the day, this cycle becomes more straightforward once they become daily schedule.

You've done a few astonishing things here, and adhering to them prompts life change. At one point, you'll supplant that large number of negative propensities with positive ones. That is the magnificence of this cycle, and I'm exceptionally eager to see your change and see what you can achieve as you push ahead on this excursion.

At last, before you go, I prescribe adhering to three guidelines for your weight reduction endeavors:

1. Focus on transient objectives. At the point when we take a gander at a drawn out objective that is excessively far away, our psyches can't zero in on it accurately. The genuine skirmish of weight reduction is battled each inch in turn, each dinner in turn, each day in turn. We're bad at zeroing in on long haul objectives. We want transient objectives since we can rapidly

see their belongings. That is the explanation we commit eating less junk food errors in any case. Transient delight overpowers our craving for long haul joy. So our recommendation is to make objectives that emphasis on the short term, similar to a particular objective for every month.

2. Start getting it on paper. Promise to record all that you eat and each time you work out. You can utilize an application, a device, or a journal. By just following what comes in and leaves your body, you will begin to consider yourself responsible. Furthermore, what's shockingly better is that errors aren't nothing to joke about when they're seen in setting. Eating a cut of pizza can feel like an outright disappointment and the demise of your eating regimen assuming that you see that solitary day. At the point when you view at it as a pattern and as a feature of three weeks of progress, it's a solitary second out of a month. It's anything but nothing to joke about. You essentially record your misstep in your diary and continue to push ahead. So promise to record what you eat, regardless of anything! Pardon yourself when you commit errors. All things considered, we want to make a record and not judge ourselves.

3. Make your objectives explicit and clear. Like that, you know precisely which objective you fizzled at, what turned out badly, and how you can keep those disappointments from rehashing. It is exclusively by gaining from your errors that you will actually want to develop, and life will keep on getting to the next level. It requires a ton of work to get thinner (and keep it off). The undertaking will endure forever.

Ideally, this book equipped you with a couple of pieces that you can use during this weight reduction venture. I hope everything works out for you!